The Silent World
of
Doctor and Patient

Jay Katz

THE FREE PRESS
A Division of Macmillan, Inc.
NEW YORK

Collier Macmillan Publishers
LONDON

To
Esta Mae

The Free Press
A Division of Macmillan, Inc.
866 Third Avenue, New York, N.Y. 10022

Collier Macmillan Canada, Inc.

First Free Press Paperback Edition 1986

Printed in the United States of America

printing number
1   2   3   4   5   6   7   8   9   10

Library of Congress Cataloging-in-Publication Data

Katz, Jay
    The silent world of doctor and patient.

    Bibliography: p.
    Includes index.
    1. Physician and patient. 2. Medicine—Decision
making—Psychological aspects. 3. Trust (Psychology)
4. Paternalism. I. Title.
R727.3.K34   1986   610.69'6   85-29405
ISBN 0-02-918760-5 (pbk.)

Contents

Acknowledgments

ABOUT A DECADE AGO, I decided to explore the interactions between physicians and patients in therapeutic settings. I wanted to examine and evaluate the authority which should be vested in physicians, patients, the medical profession, and the state in the conduct and supervision of medical therapy. Initially, I had no idea that these explorations would take me as far as they eventually did. It took time before I appreciated fully the oddity of physicians' insistence that patients follow doctors' orders. During my socialization as a physician I had been taught to accept the idea of doctors' Aesculapian authority over patients. When I began to doubt this authority, that was the moment when the book began to take shape in my mind.

My varied experiences and explorations that ultimately have led me to conclude that physicians and patients must share the burdens of decision are reflected throughout the book. Here I would like to acknowledge the profound influence on my writing of the setting in which I have worked and the people who have assisted me.

One of the good fortunes of anyone who teaches at Yale Law School is the opportunity, deeply embedded in the ethos of our school, to examine new ideas with students prior to writing about them, even though the study of such ideas may require offering seminars that are not traditionally part of the law school curriculum. The freedom to explore uncharted areas, of which this book is one example—not only in the privacy of one's office but also in the more public arena of the classroom—has made my life at Yale Law School an intellectually rewarding experience that after twenty-six years I still find exhilarating and hard to believe.

Thus, I would like to reverse the custom, so common in prefaces, of thanking the Dean last for "his generous support." Instead, I begin my acknowledgments with Dean Harry H. Wellington during whose tenure this book was conceived and written. I thank him not only because he was most generous in his personal encouragement and financial support of my work but also because as Dean he symbolizes what the Yale Law School has always sought to provide: a congenial atmosphere for the pursuit of scholarship according to its faculty's individual tastes. I doubt whether I could have written this book in many other settings. I am most grateful to the institution—its deans, colleagues, and students—where I have felt so happily at home for such a long time.

A good institution attracts good students. I am immensely indebted to my students. In seminar after seminar these intellectually gifted and concerned young women and men have enlightened and challenged me; they have been invaluable collaborators. Those of my former students who will read this book will surely pause often and recall that issues they had raised are reflected in what I have written. I can only acknowledge my intellectual and emotional debt to them for having joined me in this book as intrepid but anonymous contributors. Were I to identify them, I would have to list hundreds of students.

Similarly, I cannot name the scores of medical colleagues and friends with whom on walks, over drinks, at conferences, or while a visiting professor at their medical schools, I have discussed the problems of physician-patient decision making. I have learned a great deal from all that these colleagues and friends have shared with me about their own experiences with patients. My own patients and other physicians' patients, who over the years have consulted me about problems they had encountered in their decision-making struggles with their doctors, have also taught me much about their experiences as patients. I am grateful to these informants for enriching the clinical dimension of my explorations.

I can only acknowledge by name those who have read and criticized various drafts of this book. Their gentle and not so gentle comments have shaped this book and I profited from their caring attention: Irene Adams, Robert S. Adams, Robert L. Arnstein, Mirjan Damaska, Victor Erlich, Harry Frankfurt, Joseph Katz, Esta Mae Katz, Reinier Kraakman, Robert J. Levine, Ernst Prelinger, Adina Schwartz, Marjery Shaw, Alan J. Weisbard, and Ellen Wertheimer. Over the years, I have talked endlessly about my work with my friend and colleague Robert A. Burt and we have influenced each other in many ways. Our personal and intellectual relationship has meant much to me.

At various stages in the preparation of the manuscript, three former students were my research assistants: Ellen Wright Clayton, Sarah Cohn, and Bruce Baker. Each in their own style prodded me to clarify my thinking, and forced me to rework and refine my arguments. I am grateful for the intensity of their intellectual support which significantly affected the book's final shape.

I thank the staff of the Yale Law School library, especially Gene Coakley, for locating hundreds of articles and books that often were hard to find. My secretary Sharon O'Connell not only learned to decipher my almost illegible script but also retyped innumerable drafts without complaint. I am grateful to her for easing my task by providing me with clean copy every morning.

Laura Wolff, my editor at The Free Press, was most insistent that I delay no longer and hand over a manuscript, but at the same time she appreciated my need of not letting it go until I had said what I wanted to say. She carried out this assignment with sensitivity and tact. Similarly, Eileen DeWald, also at The Free Press, was most supportive during the arduous process of getting the manuscript ready for publication. The graceful copyediting of the manuscript by Debbie Weiss improved its clarity. Nancy Herington prepared a superb index. I thank them all.

During the book's long gestation period, I received financial support from many sources. I am most appreciative of this support which allowed me to pursue my work with more total absorption than would otherwise have been possible. An early grant from The Kayden Foundation and the Elizabeth K. Dollard Fund permitted me to spend a year doing research in preparation for writing this book. The simultaneous awards of a John Simon Guggenheim Memorial Foundation Fellowship and a NIH Grant (#00058), a Special Scientific Project Grant sponsored by the National Library of Medicine, gave me another full year, free of any teaching obligations, to write the first drafts of the entire book. Over the years, a grant from the Commonwealth Fund Program in Law, Science, and Medicine at Yale Law School allowed me to develop seminars that explored many of the issues discussed in this volume. While a guest of the Rockefeller Foundation at its Bellagio Study and Conference Center I reedited chapters of the book in a setting of indescribable beauty and comfort, yet also most conducive to scholarly work.

Finally, let me express my gratitude for the loving encouragement that I have received from my family: my brothers Joseph and Norman, Esta Mae, Sally, Daniel, and Amy. Their faith in me and that of many identified and anonymous friends, colleagues, and students has been great. I can only hope that this book, whether they agree with it or not, conveys the seriousness of purpose which throughout guided its writing.

New Haven, Connecticut
October 20, 1983

Preface to the

Paperback Edition

This book is about patients and doctors and how they make decisions. In writing it, I wanted to document two facts. First, patients by and large have been, and continue to be, excluded from participation in the decisions that vitally affect their lives. Second, inviting patients to share the burdens of decision is an inordinately difficult assignment which physicians cannot undertake until they have learned how to extend such an invitation.

Critics of my book have raised three major, albeit contradictory, objections: (1) patients are unable and unwilling to make medical decisions; (2) physician-patient decision making has sufficiently improved so that a reform of current practices is no longer a pressing concern; and (3) patient participation in decision making will impose intolerable economic costs on an already too costly medical system.

I want to take this opportunity to respond to these criticisms. Let me begin by adding one story to the many I relate throughout the book. Stories have a way of testifying to existing problems and facilitating analysis.

Recently, a renowned non-medical university professor, whom I know well, was hospitalized after his first acute gall bladder attack. His surgeon recommended immediate removal of the gall bladder. He did not mention any alternative treatments to his patient. My friend sought my advice. After talking with his surgeon and another knowledgeable medical colleague, I told my friend that removal of the gall bladder was not mandatory. We then discussed his two options—removal or non-removal of the gall bladder—and their consequences: He might not suffer another attack, but if he did, it could pass uneventfully once again. On the other hand, he was now in good physical condition, in the hands of an excellent surgeon, and if he were to worry unduly about a future recurrence, removal of the gall bladder would quiet his anxieties once and for all. Also, if the operation eventually became mandatory, competent medical help might not be available (my colleague travelled frequently to distant lands) and he also might not be in as good a physical condition to withstand the operation as he was now. All these uncertainties, including the possibility of major, although rare, surgical and post-operative complications, I discussed with him. My underlying message was: *The* right decision was *his* decision.

He understood me well. (Before relating the end of the story, I should add that my friend's scholarly and personal life attests to the high value he places on full, honest disclosure and individual choice). While thanking me with accustomed generosity, his speech became increasingly inaudible. To hear him, I had to lean over his bed, moving my ear ever closer to his lips. In a whisper, he concluded with a question: "But Jay, don't I have to do what my surgeon wants me to do?"

My friend's surgeon did not attempt to apprise his patient of available options. Nor did he try to ascertain whether my friend wished to submit to or postpone the operation, even though both were medically sound alternatives. Physicians all too rarely discuss alternatives despite the fact that, thanks to the remarkable advances of modern medicine, many alternatives are available, each with its own benefits and risks, and each affecting quality of life in decisive and often irreversible ways. In particular, the alternative of no treatment and watchful waiting—as was the option in this instance—often is not explored with patients.

Physicians do not invite patients to make decisions with them out of deeply ingrained convictions that patients are unable and unwilling to share the burdens of decision making with their doctors. The attributions of incapacity and unwillingness deserve separate consideration.

My friend's surgeon assumed, without inquiry, that his patient was incapable of contributing to the decision of whether or not to proceed with surgery. The idea of consulting with his patient did not occur to him because he, like many physicians, may have believed that patients are too frightened and too regressed to decide with him, that patients must be treated like children in need of parenting. With childlike incapacity assumed, he could not learn whether his patient's preferences might have altered the recommendation. Thus, both were locked into a decision which had not been thought through by either.

Moreover, the surgeon may have subscribed to the widely help professional belief that medicine's esoteric knowledge cannot be understood by patients, that to acquire medical wisdom requires prolonged study and clinical experience which patients do not possess. Such contentions overlook the fact that the esoteric knowledge physicians need to acquire for purposes of diagnosis and treatment is quite different from the knowledge physicians need to communicate to their patients for purposes of decision making. My friend's case demonstrates that he could have been given sufficient and comprehensible information about his medical condition to permit him to make a significant contribution to the ultimate choice.

The surgeon may also have believed, as physicians commonly do, that explanation is unnecessary, if not irrelevant, because doctor and patient have an identity of interest in medical matters. In this view, no conflict exists between them; one can decide for the other. Yet as my friend's situation also demonstrates, the objectives of health and cure can be pursued in a variety of ways, each with its attendant risks and benefits. Physicians' personal and professional experience and preferences may dictate one course; patients' needs, expectations, and preferences another one. Had the surgeon invited my friend's views about whether or not to operate, they would soon have discovered together whether the patient was capable of making a choice. If incapable, my friend probably would have acknowledged his incapacity and conferred on his doctor the authority to proceed according to the latter's best judgment.

There is another problem. Patients, in being deprived of basic information about their conditions and alternative treatment options, are in no position to raise the quesions they may want to ask but cannot clearly formulate. When they then appear confused, stupid, embarrassed, and tongue-tied, doctors (and often patients too) view such behavior as evidence of incapacity. Thus, incapacity, all too readily assumed and, in turn, fostered by physicians, becomes a self-fulfilling prophesy.

It is equally unclear whether my friend was willing or unwilling to decide himself whether to undergo surgery. His final question highlights the awe, deference, and fear with which patients approach their physicians. The idea of questioning, not to speak of refusing, a doctor's order is difficult for patients to contemplate, if not out of habit then out of other concerns. For example, patients often feel compelled to surrender their right to ask probing questions out of fear of offending their doctors and out of guilt about imposing on their time. However distorted these concerns are, they guide patients' interactions with their doctors and, unless vigorously opposed by physicians, they will affect the phyician-patient dialogue in self-fulfilling ways.

Lest I be misunderstood, let me emphasize that I do not question that some, perhaps many, patients may wish their doctors to decide for them. However, whether the compliance ultimately expresses patients' wishes can only be ascertained if doctors first inform their patients that they are willing to take the time to make decisions together, and that they are prepared to explain what is at stake. Without such an offer, neither doctors, nor for that matter patients, can be certain whether compliance was compelled by physicians' conduct that patients felt unprepared to oppose. In the latter case, both often learn about such misgivings too late when patients turn away from their doctors with bitter disappointment or file malpractice suits.

Doctors cannot know how many patients are unable or unwilling to participate in decision making until they radically change their perceptions of patients, assist patients in altering their perceptions of their doctors, and learn to speak with patients in new and unaccustomed ways. Put another way, to learn whether patients are able and willing to make decisions jointly requires *first* that doctors take responsibility for altering traditional patterns of interacting with their patients; only *then* can patients be expected to assume the responsibility of informing their doctors that they wish to have a voice in decision making.

My critics' second contention that significant improvements have occurred in the physician-patient dialogue dismisses too lightly the central arguments of my book: (1) that meaningful collaboration between physicians and patients cannot become a reality until physicians have learned how to treat their patients not as children but as the adults they are; how to distinguish between their ideas of the best treatment and their patients' ideas of what is best; and how to acknowledge to their patients (and often to themselves as well) their ignorance and uncertainties about diagnosis, treatment, and prognosis; and (2) that medical educators have failed to prepare future physicians for the responsibilities that shared decision making imposes. While the education of physicians for technical competence is at a remarkably high level, their education for shared decision-making competence is deficient. Medical educators need to appreciate more than they do that learning how to converse with patients is as difficult a task as learning about diseases, their patho-physiology, diagnosis, and treatment. As Franz Kafka observed, "[t]o prescribe pills is easy but to reach an understanding with people is very hard."

Finally, my friend's story illustrates that it does not take undue time to explain available options to patients. Time costs have frequently been invoked as economically inimical to shared decision making. I do not believe that time costs are either that serious an impediment or the real culprit.

Surely in surgical interventions, the high fees charged provide surgeons with adequate compensation for also taking the time to make themselves better understood. Moreover, in all elective procedures, as in my friend's case, no surgical intervention is always a viable alternative. Thus, if the alternative of no intervention were more fully explored with patients, some might very well decide against the recommended treatment with consequent considerable savings to the health care system. Of course, individual physicians would be deprived of a fee, but that is another matter.

Unfamiliarity with how to talk, unwillingness to talk, embarrassment about admitting ignorance and uncertainty, and loss of income are greater obstacles than time costs. If I am wrong and the cost of conversation proves to be considerable, then physicians must acknowledge that such costs undermine disclosure and consent and, therefore, shared decision making remains a charade. Alternatively, if time costs need to be taken seriously, doctors can at least try to identify those interventions—e.g., elective procedures or treatments accompanied by serious morbidities and mortalities—for which full disclosure becomes imperative out of respect for good patient care.

Let me conclude by expressing the hope that patients will read this book and demand to be treated differently. Being a physician and teacher, I also hope that medical students will study it carefully and critically. They, unlike my generation, may be more willing to move medicine into a new age in which the benefits and risks of medicine's spectacular advances will be accepted or rejected by their patients only after respectful and mutual deliberation. At a minimum, a younger generation of scientifically trained physicians may be more inclined to experiment with new ways of interacting with patients in order to find out whether the practice of medicine will prove to be more rewarding to doctors and patients if both share the burdens of decision making. In this age of depersonalizing medical science and acrimonious malpractice litigation, the need for such interaction is even more compelling; for physicians must learn whether a radically different dialogue with patients will restore confidence in the humanity of a great profession.

Introduction

THIS IS A BOOK about doctors and patients by a physician who has spent most of his professional life teaching in a school of law. Being both an insider and an outsider to the worlds of medicine and law has perhaps given me the perspective to describe and to comment on how doctors and patients arrive at decisions that have such a significant impact on patients' well-being. Throughout the ages, physicians have consistently excluded patients from sharing with them the burdens of decision; only in recent decades have judges begun to prod doctors to be somewhat more attentive to patients' decision-making rights and needs. Thus, it is not surprising that this latest controversy between the worlds of medicine and law has created new misunderstanding, confusion, and acrimony.

This book's ultimate purpose is to initiate a more enlightened debate about the respective rights, duties, and needs of physicians and patients in their intimate, anxiety-producing, and fateful encounters with one another. While I shall be quite critical of doctors' interactions with patients, I do not mean to condemn. Many of the problems explored in this book have not been pursued in any depth before. Thus condemnation, if ever of value, is at least premature in this instance. Moreover, physicians deserve better. They have made significant contributions to the well-being of mankind. No other profession has done more. But I shall not dwell on these remarkable accomplishments and to that extent the book is one-sided. Instead, its focus is on one facet of medical practice—the microcosm of decision making between physicians and patients.

At least since Hippocratic days, patients have been asked to trust their physicians without question. But only in recent years have doctors been asked to trust patients by conversing with them about medical options and soliciting their views on how to proceed. The idea that conversation will lead to mutually satisfactory decisions is not one of human beings' most abiding convictions. Therefore, to ask physicians and patients to get to know themselves and each other better through conversation will encounter resistance. What has been true for the evolution of mankind has been equally true for the progress of medicine: We have spared no effort to make better tools but we have paid little attention to learning how to communicate better with one another.

Physicians' persistent and relentless demand that patients trust their doctors or, as Talcott Parsons has put it, that patients "follow doctors' orders,"[1] should have alerted doctors to the fact that patients may not trust them, or that they trust them only with profound reservations. Social science studies on patient compliance have consistently supported the depressing conclusion that a great many patients do not comply with their doctors' prescriptions and that their physicians are largely unaware of such practices.[2] The newly imposed legal requirement of informed consent—the dual obligations to inform patients and to obtain their consent—is only modern proof that trust in the professional is no longer viewed as sufficient protection of the integrity of the physician-patient relationship. Instead, the idea of informed consent suggests that trust must be earned through conversation.

It takes the skills of a novelist to speak insightfully about the interrelationship between trust and conversation. In his book, *Cancer Ward*, Solzhenitsyn highlighted problems of trust and conversation in his depiction of the encounter between Doctor Ludmilla Afanasyevna, a radiation therapist, and Oleg Kostoglotov, her patient. Kostoglotov suffered from a malignancy, for the moment in partial remission. Afanasyevna wanted to continue to treat the tumor aggressively but Kostoglotov demurred. He had had enough of painful treatments. What made conversation between them virtually impossible was his precious secret that he could not share with Afanasyevna—his intention to treat himself as soon as he could escape from the hospital with "a secret medicine, a mandrake root from Issyk Kul."[3]

He knew that he could not trust her with this piece of information, and not because she would not have talked with him about it. In fact, they might very well have debated for a while the relative efficacy of radiation, chemotherapy, and mandrake roots. Eventually, however, the question would have arisen: "Who decides?" Earlier in the interview, in response to Kostoglotov's challenge of doctors' rights to make unilateral decisions on behalf of patients, Afanasyevna had given to this question a troubled, though unequivocal, answer: "But doctors *are* entitled to that right—doctors above all. Without that right there'd be no such thing as medicine!"

This puts it starkly. Yet what is one to make of Afanasyevna's fears that with conversation that respects the rights and needs of both parties to assume the burdens of decision "there'd be no such thing as medicine"? Is she merely giving voice to one of those paralyzing fears that so frequently surface whenever the old order is threatened, or is she telling us that mutual conversations between doctor and patient will radically change medical practices as we know them?

If Afanasyevna is correct that doctors are "entitled to that right," then patients must continue to trust them silently. For conversation to be meaningful, both parties must be entitled to make decisions and to have their choices treated with respect. Trust, based on blind faith—on passive surrender to oneself or to another—must be distinguished from trust that is earned after having first acknowledged to oneself and then shared with the other what one knows and does not know about the decision to be made. Although such mutual trust is difficult to embrace and to sustain, it is important to strive for it.

The proponents of informed consent and patient self-determination have insufficiently appreciated that trusting oneself and others to become aware of the certainties and uncertainties that surround the practice of medicine, and to integrate them with one's hopes, fears, and realistic expectations, are inordinately difficult tasks. They are among the tasks, however, that fidelity to disclosure and consent requires physicians and patients to undertake. The opponents of informed consent, on the other hand, have insufficiently appreciated that disclosure and consent do not abolish trust. Disclosure and consent only banish unilateral, blind trust; they make mutual trust possible for the first time.

Historically, surrender to silent and blind trust in the physician was to a considerable extent compelled by the state of the art—by medicine's uncertainties that could not be explicated easily. Only during the last 150 years, thanks to the unprecedented advances in medical science, have physicians begun to acquire the intellectual sophistication and experimental tools to distinguish more systematically between knowledge and ignorance, between what they know, do not know, and what remains conjectural. These so recently acquired capacities have permitted physicians to consider for the first time whether to entrust their certainties and uncertainties to their patients. Disclosure and consent now are viable alternatives to keeping patients in the dark and making decisions on their behalf. Without the emergence of medical science, the legal doctrine of informed consent probably could not have been promulgated.

Judges' intention behind the doctrine of informed consent was to give patients a greater voice in decision making, to improve the climate of conversation between physicians and patients. The courts largely undercut this intention, however, with profound reservations that revealed their distrust of patients' capacities to make their own decisions. Thus the doctrine of informed consent allowed physicians to retain considerable "discretion" to make choices for patients. The doctrine has suffered from judges' convictions that doctors know better than patients what is good for patients. The promise to endow patients with the right to "thorough-going self-determination,"[4] which was to be the basis of the informed consent doctrine, remains largely unfulfilled. To distinguish between what judges have done and what they have aspired to, one must draw sharp distinctions between the *legal* doctrine, as promulgated by judges, and the *idea* of informed consent, based on a commitment to individual self-determination.

This book will offer contemporary and historical evidence that patients' participation in decision making is an idea alien to the ethos of medicine. The humane care that physicians have extended to patients throughout the ages rarely has been based on the humaneness of consensual understanding; rather it has been based on the humaneness of services silently rendered. It is the time-honored professional belief in the virtue of silence, based on ancient notions of a need for faith, reassurance, and hope, that the idea of informed consent seeks to question.

History has its reasons. It cannot be accidental that the principles of medical ethics have never commanded physicians and their patients to get to know and understand one another so that they can make decisions jointly. We need to inquire why physicians have been so insistent in their demand that all authority be vested in one party—the doctor.

One important reason for this insistence is physicians' unfamiliarity with and embarrassment over conversing with patients about medical ignorance and uncertainties that can so decisively affect choice of treatment. This problem has become more acute during this century, due to physicians' increased capacities to distinguish knowledge from ignorance and uncertainty. Revelation of such uncertainties is difficult and disquieting. Learning to live more comfortably with uncertainty, however, has also been impeded by other strongly held, although largely unexamined, professional beliefs: that patients are unable to tolerate awareness of uncertainty, and that faith in professionals and their prescriptions makes a significant contribution to the optimal treatment of disease.

In the light of these and other problems it is not surprising that doctors are most reluctant to share authority with patients and instead insist that patients follow doctors' orders. Authority so conceived and exercised seems to make doctors' lives easier. At the same time, the considerable strain that the usurpation of solitary responsibility over patients' fate imposes on physicians has not received the attention it deserves.

The delegation of such sweeping authority to physicians has engendered considerable concerns among patients and the general public about abuse of authority. Doctors have tried to allay these concerns by pointing to the common objectives of doctor and patient. Moreover, doctors have emphasized their abiding commitment to altruistic service and the protection it provides to patients. Both contentions, however, are flawed.

To be sure, physicians and patients are united in the common pursuit of restoring patients to "healthy" life. Since that objective rarely can be fully achieved, however, it remains an ambiguous one. To the extent it can be achieved it is attainable by many different and uncertain routes, each with its own benefits and costs. In the absence of any one clear road to well-being, identity of interest cannot be assumed, and consensus on goals, let alone on which paths to follow, can only be accomplished through conversation. Two distinct and separate parties interact with one another—not one mind (the physician's), not one body (the patient's), but two minds and two bodies. Moreover, both parties bring conflicting motivations and interests to their encounters. Professional considerations, personal value judgments, and self-interest decisively influence physicians' pronouncements. Personal values, considerations of life style, and other competing preferences influence patients' choices. Conflicts within and between the parties are inevitable. Silent altruism alone cannot resolve these conflicting tensions.

Thus, informed consent's implicit demand for joint decision making confronts the painful realization that even in their most intimate relationships, human beings remain strangers to one another. One can only know and understand *another* to a limited extent. But the problem runs even deeper. One can only understand *oneself* to a limited extent. The latter impediment powerfully reinforces the former, making it even more difficult to know another.

Physicians and patients are not exempt from this human tragedy. Its pervasive impact on all human encounters contradicts one of the most basic and revered professional dogmas: that doctors can be totally trusted because they act only "in their patients' best interests." This dogma only compounds the tragedy by assuming an identity of interests and brushing aside the necessity of clarifying differences in expectations and objectives through conversation. Particularly in today's medical world, where so many treatment options are available—each with its own benefits and risks, and each championed by physicians depending on their personal and professional preferences—the conflicting interests must be better identified. In this age of specialization, professional preferences can create more problems than ever, for a patient's "choice" of treatment may be affected decisively by the kind of specialist he has happened to consult first.

Sharing with patients the burdens of decision will also stimulate interest in finding answers to another question: How personal can the physician-patient relationship become and how depersonalized must it remain? A conversation between a senior physician and a medical intern illustrates this problem.[5] The senior physician asked the intern how much he knew about "patients as human beings." The question led to a rather nonproductive exchange that the intern ended abruptly with the exasperated comment: "I cannot answer your questions. You're interested in patients, I'm interested in the disease in the body in the bed." An unbridgeable gap was created between the intern and the senior physician because they had neglected to explore first questions such as: What can and must the intern and the senior physician learn about a patient in order not to reduce him to a mere inhuman object? In what ways are patients the same or different from other human beings encountered in intimate, non-professional settings? To what extent need a patient remain "a body in the bed" in the minds of the intern and senior physician?

Furthermore, shared decision making challenges professional convictions that patients are too ignorant about medical matters and too anxious about being ill to make decisions on their own behalf. These deeply held beliefs raise questions about patients' capacities for autonomous conduct. Patients' alleged limitations for autonomous decision making, however, must be evaluated against similar limitations in physicians' capacities for decision making as well as the contributions that physicians make to undermining patients' capacities for autonomous conduct by treating them largely as incompetent children. I shall attempt to rescue the concept of autonomy from the abstractions that have governed its application and to place it instead more firmly in the reality of human psychology and the living context of physician-patient interactions.

The problems of informed consent, or better, of greater patient participation in the medical decision-making process, require an exploration of the historical evolution of medicine and the medical profession, law, the psychology of physicians and patients, and the state of the art and science of medicine. This exploration will demonstrate that a commitment to the idea of informed consent is not easy. Taking such a commitment seriously requires, prior to implementation, a careful scholarly analysis of the complexities of physician-patient decision making. These problems deserve study and their in-depth analysis must be extended beyond where I leave off. The more I reflect about informed consent the more I appreciate how many additional leads need to be pursued. In this book I have been unable to explore any to their depth. Instead, I have tried to identify as many issues as possible and to pursue them for some distance.

The study of informed consent can also be viewed as an opportunity to reestablish a rightful place for the ancient practice of the art of medicine. The practice of medicine's art has been given short shrift in this age of science, in the expectation that treatment only requires silent scalpels, wordless monitors, and mute pharmacological agents. The public has begun to rebel against such treatment, however, and physicians also have begun to wonder how to "humanize" doctors by "humanizing" their training.

Francis Peabody concluded his famous lecture on "The Care of the Patient" with these moving words:

> [t]he good physician knows his patients through and through, and his knowledge is bought dearly. Time, sympathy, and understanding must be lavishly dispensed, but the reward is to be found in that personal bond which forms the greatest satisfaction of the practice of medicine. One of the essential qualities of the clinician is interest in humanity, for the secret of the care of the patient is in caring for the patient.[6]

If "interest in humanity" is an essential professional quality, and if it defines, as I believe it does, the art of medicine, it must be taught and learned as thoroughly as medicine's science is now being taught and learned.

This book seeks to make a contribution to this objective by demonstrating how difficult, although intellectually worthwhile and emotionally intriguing, such an undertaking can prove to be. If seriously pursued, it may lead to another Flexner report.[7] The first one led to drastic revisions in medical students' clinical and theoretical education. The new one may recommend that medical students become better educated for the practice of the art of medicine. Implementation of such a proposal will require a greater commitment than merely admonishing physicians not to neglect their art and, once having said that, to neglect its teaching in the science-stuffed curriculum.

It is dangerous nonsense to assert that in the practice of their art and science physicians can rely on their benevolent intentions, their abilities to judge what is the right thing to do, or their capacities for conducting their rounds with humanity, patience, prudence, and wisdom—all supposedly acquired through on-the-job training. It is not that easy. Medicine is a complex profession and the interactions between physicians and patients are also complex. To practice the art of medicine responsibly, requires as committed and as rigorous a study as learning its science demands.

What is true for physicians is equally true for patients. They, too, must learn that it is in their best interests to appreciate better than they now do that the practice of medicine is to a great extent still shrouded in uncertainty and that its practitioners, however competent and dedicated, are also fallible human beings. Only then will patients learn to question their doctors and to ask questions of their doctors.

Above all, physicians and patients must learn to converse with one another. Meaningful conversation, however, requires that both are also prepared to trust each other. Powerful obstacles stand in the path of trust and conversation. This book seeks to identify the obstacles and clear a path on which physicians and patients can travel with mutual appreciation that the burdens of decision rest on both their shoulders.

I

Physicians and Patients: A History of Silence

IN THIS CHAPTER I intend to document that disclosure and consent, except in the most rudimentary fashion, are obligations alien to medical thinking and practice. Disclosure in medicine has served the function of getting patients to "consent" to what physicians wanted them to agree to in the first place. "Good" patients follow doctor's orders without question. Therefore, disclosure becomes relevant only with recalcitrant patients. Since they are "bad" and "ungrateful," one does not need to bother much with them. Hippocrates once said, "Life is short, the Art long, Opportunity fleeting, Experiment treacherous, Judgment difficult. The physician must be ready, not only to do his duty himself, but also to secure the co-operation of the patient, of the attendants and of externals."[1] These were, and still are, the lonely obligations of physicians: to wrestle as best they can with life, art, opportunity, experiment and judgment. Sharing with patients the vagaries of available opportunities, however perilous or safe, or the rationale underlying judgments, however difficult or easy, is not part of the Hippocratic task. For doing that, the Art is too long and Life too short.

Physicians have always maintained that patients are only in need of caring custody. Doctors felt that in order to accomplish that objective they were obligated to attend to their patients' physical and emotional needs and to do so on their own authority, without consulting with their patients about the decisions that needed to be made. Indeed, doctors intuitively believed that such consultations were inimical to good patient care. The idea that patients may also be entitled to liberty, to sharing the burdens of decision with their doctors, was never part of the ethos of medicine. Being unaware of the idea of patient liberty, physicians did not address the possible conflict between notions of custody and liberty. When, however, in recent decades courts were confronted with allegations that professionals had deprived citizen-patients of freedom of choice, the conflict did emerge. Anglo-American law has, at least in theory, a long-standing tradition of preferring liberty over custody; and however much judges tried to sidestep law's preferences and to side with physicians' traditional beliefs, the conflict remained and has ever since begged for a resolution.

The legal doctrine of informed consent is only 25 years old. Through it, judges sought to protect patients' right to greater freedom of choice by obligating physicians "to disclose and explain to the patient in language as simple as necessary the nature of the ailment, the nature of the proposed treatment, the probability of success or of alternatives, and perhaps the risks of unfortunate results and unforeseen conditions within the body."[2] In Chapter III I shall make much of the fact that the judges who gave physicians these marching orders did not tell them where or how far to march, or how deeply to infiltrate the newly discovered world, where in the words of one court, "the patient's right of self-decision shapes the boundaries of the duty to reveal."[3] For now, let me highlight another fact that will always loom important in the history of physician-patient relations: the pronouncements of the common law judges, although limited in scope, penetrated for the first time the mystery, isolation, and loneliness of professional decision making.

The legal doctrine remained limited in scope, in part, because judges believed or wished to believe that their pronouncements on informed consent gave legal force to what good physicians customarily did; therefore they felt that they could defer to the disclosure practices of "reasonable medical practitioners."[4] Judges did not appreciate how deeply rooted the tradition of silence was and thus did not recognize the revolutionary, alien implications of their appeal for patient "self-determination." In fact, precisely because of the appeal's strange and bewildering novelty, physicians misinterpreted it as being more far-reaching than courts intended it to be.

Physicians did not realize how much their opposition to informed consent was influenced by suddenly encountering obligations divorced from their history, their clinical experience, or medical education. Had they appreciated that even the doctrine's modest appeal to patient self-determination represented a radical break with medical practices, as transmitted from teacher to student during more than two thousand years of recorded medical history, they might have been less embarrassed by standing so unpreparedly, so nakedly before this new obligation. They might then perhaps have realized that their silence had been until most recently a historical necessity, dictated not only by the inadequacy of medical knowledge but also by physicians' incapacity to discriminate between therapeutic effectiveness based on their actual physical interventions and benefits that must be ascribed to other causes. They might also have argued that the practice of silence was part of a long and venerable tradition that deserved not to be dismissed lightly. They might at least have pleaded for time, because before they could embrace the unaccustomed obligation to talk with their patients, many problems required intensive study. None of this happened. Instead passive-aggressive defensiveness, acrimony, and confusion have marked the early history of the age of informed consent. The physician-patient dialogue, now a mixture of proffered and withheld information, has become even more opaque; surely it is not based on the idea of shared decision making.

In subsequent chapters I shall explore the many reasons for physicians', indeed for all professionals', opposition to the idea of informed consent. In what follows here I wish to convey the stark silence that throughout medical history has been the hallmark of physicians' attitudes toward patients' participation in medical decision making. When I speak of silence I do not mean to suggest that physicians have not talked to their patients at all. Of course, they have conversed with patients about all kinds of matters, but they have not, except inadvertently, employed words to invite patients' participation in sharing the burden of making joint decisions.

Ancient Medicine

The earliest records of Western medicine, in what they reveal about physician-patient dialogue, document the silence. The Hippocratic Oath makes no reference to physicians' obligation to converse with patients. The specified duties were of a different nature: "[to] follow that system of regimen which, according to my ability and judgment, I consider for the benefit of my patients, and abstain from whatever is deleterious and mischievous."[5] Indeed, the only explicit advice on conversation within the Hippocratic Corpus speaks against disclosure. In *Decorum*, Hippocrates admonished physicians to

> [p]erform [these duties] calmly and adroitly, concealing most things from the patient while you are attending to him. Give necessary orders with cheerfulness and serenity, turning his attention away from what is being done to him; sometimes reprove sharply and emphatically, and sometimes comfort with solicitude and attention, revealing nothing of the patient's future or present condition.[6]

Plato, whose Dialogues give a reasonably complete account of medical practice in classical Greece, did not suggest that the lively interactions among the participants in his Dialogues should become a model for the interactions between physician and patient. Dialogue surely was not indicated for the medical treatment of slaves. Such patients should never be talked to individually or be allowed to talk much about their complaints. Instead the doctor "prescribes what mere experience suggests, as if he had exact knowledge; and [once] he has given his orders, like a tyrant, he rushes off."[7]

The philosophy underlying the treatment of slaves subtly infiltrated the treatment of other citizens, for the treatment of "the free but poor" was not very different. While they were not to be treated "tyrannically," they were to be worked over resolutely with "an emetic or a purge or cautery or the knife," for they could not be expected to heed a physician's advice to undergo a complicated course of treatment. They have "no time to be ill"[8]; therefore it was a waste of time to talk with them.

While studying the treatment of "the free but poor" in classical Greece, I was reminded of a conversation with a distinguished French nephrologist. Our conversation testifies to the persistence of ancient attitudes and prescriptions into modern times. Immediately prior to our meeting the nephrologist had examined a French peasant who lived some 40 miles outside of Paris and suffered from chronic renal failure. The condition was a rapidly progressive one and would soon lead to death unless the patient were placed on renal dialysis. Yet the patient was not offered this option. Instead, he was told that no medical treatment existed that would help him. When I asked the nephrologist why he had concealed the alternative of dialysis from his patient, he reacted with surprise, as if the answer were self-evident: "To say more would have been cruel. Peasants do not adjust well to a permanent move to a large city." Dialysis would have required a permanent relocation. His words echoed those of Plato who millenia earlier, after commenting that poor patients have no time to be ill, went on to say that the poor patient

> sees no good in a life which is spent in nursing his disease to the neglect of his customary employment; and therefore bidding good-bye to this sort of physician, he resumes his ordinary habits, and either gets well and lives and does his business, or if his constitution fails, he dies and has no more troubles.[9]

But who, in either Plato's day or our own, bids good-bye to whom? Is it the patient, as Plato implied, or is it the physician as my modern example suggests? The interrelationship between silence and abandonment will preoccupy us throughout this book.

Plato also described the treatment of a third group of patients, "the free and rich." Their care was more delicate and individualized than that of the slaves and the poor; the doctor "enters into discourse with the patient and with his friends, and is at once getting information from the sick man, and also instructing him as far as he is able."[10] However, conversation did not serve the objective of inviting patient participation in decision making. Instead, the prescribed "enlightenment" of patients served the purposes of preventive medicine (once patients learned how their suffering came about, they might be able to control the cause), of more accurate diagnosis (patients' accurate knowledge of themselves helped diagnosis), or gaining patients' confidence through verbal persuasion. A good doctor, Plato wrote, will not prescribe for a "free and rich" patient until he has first convinced him that the treatment will be effective. Only "when [at last] he has brought the patient more and more under his persuasive influences and set him on the road to health, he attempts to effect a cure."[11]

Physicians of ancient Greece were keenly aware of the importance of confidence and faith in the treatment of disease. A call for shared decision making would have puzzled them. Such an appeal would have seemed to them unnecessary, counterproductive, and therefore contraindicated. They would have considered it unnecessary because they viewed doctor and patient as united through *philia*, friendship, which made their objectives one and the same.[12] "The sick man loves the physicians because he is sick,"[13] said Plato. Hippocrates in a famous passage declared, "Where there is *philanthropia* (love of man), there is also *philotechnia* (love of the art [of healing])."[14] Unity through *philia* in Greek days has a modern counterpart: "identity of interests." Whatever the label, this notion makes conversation unnecessary, if not irrelevant. There is no "other" who requires an explanation, for both want the same things: recovery and cure. The dangers inherent in obliterating the separate identities of physician and patient, which neither in health nor in sickness can ever become one, were not, and still are not, sufficiently appreciated.

The ancient Greeks would have considered patient participation counterproductive because instilling confidence and dispelling doubts required persuading patients by any available means of the correctness of doctors' prescriptions. Greek physicians believed that physicians' effectiveness depended on *philanthropia* that, in turn, kindled in patients *philotechnia* (love of the [medical] art), with both states of mind contributing greatly to speedy recovery. To accomplish that objective—which after all is what the practice of medicine is all about—Socrates believed that physicians had to be aware of "the healing effects of fair words."[15] Conversations between physicians and "free and rich" patients were not in the service of making patients participants in decision making, but rather were meant to reinforce therapeutic effectiveness. According to Hippocrates, a patient would think a physician to be the worst doctor in the world "if he does not promise to cure what is curable and to cure what is incurable."[16]

In the ancient Greeks' view, cooperation between physician and patient was important not for the sake of sharing decision-making burdens but for the sake of friendship that, in turn, led to trust, obedience and then to cure. Centuries later the great Spanish physician Gregorio Marañon, had this progression in mind when, echoing his Hippocratic ancestors, he admonished patients, "obey your doctor and you start getting well."[17] A commitment to trust and obedience did not encourage explanation, particularly since explanations would reveal the uncertainties inherent in the art and science of medicine, creating a state of mind believed to be inimical to cure.

Medieval Medicine

The ethical legacy of Hippocratic physicians exerted a powerful influence on medical practices from ancient times to the present. For example, the medical historian Mary Welborn traced most ethical principles preserved in the works of fourteenth century medical writers to classical manuscripts, and particularly those in the Hippocratic Corpus.[18] The remarkably unchanged influence of Greek medical ethics on Arabic and Western medical practice, at least until most recently, should make one pause and reflect on the reasons for this astonishing fact before suggesting and expecting any change in the ethical conduct of physicians.

From the decline of the Greek city states to the 18th century, no major primary or secondary documents on medical ethics that I consulted, with a few minor exceptions, reveal even a remote awareness of a need to discuss anything with patients that relates to their participation in decision making. Conversations with patients served purposes of offering comfort, reassurance and hope, and of inducing patients to take the cure. Achievement of these objectives demanded an emphasis on the need to be authoritative, manipulative, and even deceitful. That emphasis was dictated less by self-serving reasons than by a wish to be helpful to patients; for without respect for medical authority, there could be no cure. As Plato had put it centuries earlier, physicians only employed lies for good and noble purposes.[19]

During this 1500 year period, interactions between physicians and patients were shaped by three interrelated beliefs: Patients must honor physicians, for they have received their authority from God; patients must have faith in their doctors; and patients must promise obedience. The three themes have at least one thing in common: they undermine both dialogue and a sharing of the burdens of decision.

The first belief is reflected in the words of the physician-author of a tenth century Brussels manuscript, who noted in a postscript, "[n]ow let us speak of the minister of nature; the physician. . . . Luke said in the Bible that it is given to physicians to be the Lord's workers. Likewise, Hippocrates said that the physician achieves just as much as God permits."[20] This is only a slight alteration of what Hippocrates had actually said in *Decorum*: "The gods are the real physicians."[21]

The close ties between physicians and God were already emphasized by ancient physicians, and only reiterated by medieval doctors of Jewish, Arabic, and Christian extraction. Thus, the Jewish physician Ben Sira wrote in the third century B.C.: "My son, should you fall sick, place yourself in the hands of a doctor, for this is his calling and God has given him of His wisdom."[22] The 9th century Arabic physician Ishāq ibn Alī-al-Ruhāwi remarked even more insistently:

> He who blames the physician discloses his ignorance; he is from the lowest class of people. . . . We have also previously said that the exalted Allah is health-giving and maintains the well-being of the healthy. He is the real physician and He taught the people that by which they keep their health and treat their illness. Then he who blames the art of medicine blames the acts of Allah, the exalted Creator.[23]

The Christian author of a late eighth century Bamberg manuscript expressed the same belief in slightly different words:

> [L]et us honor the physicians so that they will help us when sick, remember [the words of Ecclesiasticus]: "Honor the physician of necessity for the Most High created him." And do not hesitate to take what potions he gives you. [H]e who does not seek medicine in time of necessity deserves the name stupid and imprudent. I say that it is wise to do well by the physician while you are well so that you will have his services in time of illness. . . .[24]

These writers, like their ancient Greek counterparts, assumed the existence of an identity of interest between physician and patient. Now God's authority, in addition to *philanthropia* and *philo-technia*, united physicians and patients in their common pursuits. The postulated intimate relationship between physicians, patients, and their God made any critical questioning of doctors' practices by patients difficult. During the Age of Faith such an encounter came close to blasphemy. Thus, not only would patients find it difficult to question their Aesculapian physicians but the latter, being anointed by God, also would disdain explaining themselves and their practices.

In medieval as well as ancient Greek days, however, the claim to Apollonian-Aesculapian authority and the demand for obedience were not merely part of a quest for authority and power. They also were based on a deeply held belief in the importance of faith for cure that authority and obedience could only strengthen. Thus, the ninth century Jewish physician Isaac Israeli wrote: "Reassure the patient and declare his safety even though you may not be certain of it, for by this you will strengthen his Nature."[25]

Faith would assure the obedience so necessary for therapeutic effectiveness. The French surgeon Henri de Mondeville addressed the interconnections between obedience and healing when he wrote:

> The surgeon . . . should promise that if the patient can endure his illness and will obey the surgeon for a short time he will soon be cured and will escape all of the dangers which have been pointed out to him; thus the cure can be brought about more easily and more quickly. . . . If the patient is defiant, seldom will the result be successful. . . .[26]

Indeed, obedience was considered to be so critical to cure that Isaac Israeli admonished physicians:

> Should the patient not submit to your discipline, and should his servants and members of his household not be diligent in following your command quickly, nor honor you as is proper, do not persevere in the treatment.[27]

Faith and obedience were every bit as important to the practice of medieval physicians as they had been in the days of Hippocrates.

Sixteenth and Seventeenth Century Medicine

These assumptions remained unquestioned in later centuries and precluded any re-evaluation of the traditional practice to withhold information from patients. Cassiodorus, a late-sixth century physician in the Ostrogothic Kingdom of Italy—to return once more to earlier days in order to demonstrate the continuity of millenia of silence—advised physicians that "the pulsing of the veins . . . reveals the patient's ailment while the urine analysis indicates it to his eye. To make things easier, do not tell the clamoring inquirer what these symptoms signify."[28] What led Cassiodorus, and other physicians before and after him, to recommend the withholding of and tampering with information was most beautifully and thoughtfully conveyed by Samuel de Sorbière, a French physician, priest and philosopher, in a work published posthumously in 1672. It carried the imposing title "Advice to a Young Physician Respecting the Way in Which He Is to Conduct Himself in the Practice of Medicine, in View of the Indifference of the Public to the Subject, and Considering the Complaints that Are Made about Physicians."[29] The book is remarkable because de Sorbière at least entertained the idea of making fuller disclosures to patients. He both favored the idea and rejected it out of hand. His ambivalence makes him a true ancestor of many modern physicians who appreciate the value of patient participation in decision making, but then introduce so many qualifications that the idea of informed consent becomes severely compromised, if not obliterated. De Sorbière's candor and openness are quite unusual. Since the book is a prototype for essentially similar writings on patient participation in decision making, it deserves to be quoted and discussed at some length:

> Too frank and candid a manner, such as I am about to describe, might not be so successful in a young physician, whose practice as yet would not warrant such an attitude. For can you imagine him, Sir, having this conversation with a patient:—"Although I am disposed to be of service to you, and will undertake your cure as an end to be hoped for, and with God's help achieve success, in order to safeguard your interests, I must tell you that medicine is a very imperfect science, that it is quite full of guesswork, that it scarcely understands its subject matter, nor is it familiar with the things employed to maintain it; that the more enlightened only feel their way in it groping amidst a thick gloom; and that after having considered

seriously all the matters which may be useful, collected all one's thoughts, examined all one's experiences, it will indeed be a wise physician who can promise relief to a poor patient." Furthermore, that he will hazard nothing new or very unusual in his case, and that if he is not cured, at least he will do all possible to make him no worse. . . .*

Having delivered himself of these remarkable confessions, de Sorbière immediately questioned the wisdom of physicians, young or old, conducting themselves in such a manner. He argued that an ignorant person would conclude that his physician possessed neither the education nor the experience that other doctors had acquired and, therefore, would seek out "another attendant who was more positive." Moreover, he observed that patients want to deceive themselves and to be deceived about the deficiencies of medicine. Therefore, "the physician runs little danger when making use of an innocent deception in promising [a patient] more than he is certain of achieving. The wise conversation of an eminent sceptic is too delicate a viand for the common mind, and it is very needful to guard against making use of it, except with the greatest care."

De Sorbière went on to describe with approval a variety of attitudes that physicians had adopted in his day to bend their patients' will to their own, such as brusqueness, urbanity, flattery, arriving in "roadsters with their green saddle-cloths, and the four footmen in similar livery," and spouting a little Latin. He suggested that physicians must behave in such ways because

[t]here is no profession which asks more of a man than medicine. [A lawyer] has only to speak eloquently for his client; and [a clergyman] has only . . . to speak in a domineering way to the conscience of his auditor. . . . [A physician, however,] speaks only about uncertain things, with which everyone thinks it is his right to be concerned, because each pretends to some power of reasoning and to some experience; which are the two wings of medicine, wings which scarcely lift it, or carry it far. Therefore, the physician has more need to be clever than the others.

He concluded that a wise physician should always have "a few doses of nonsense to bestow." For example, de Sorbière had little

*Reprinted with permission of The Johns Hopkins University Press from 24 *Bulletin of the History of Medicine* 255–287 (1950).

faith in the diagnostic value of inspecting urine or feeling the pulse—accepted and expected medical practices in his time—but he argued in favor of accommodating oneself to "the credulity of ignorant people, who are curious to know [through such means] the conditions and the results of an illness."

De Sorbière was of two minds, however. He also hoped that the discourse between physician and patient might eventually evolve in new directions. He spoke forcefully about his hopes at the very end of his book in an imaginary monologue addressed to an intelligent patient on a first visit:

> Sir, if you have the intention of not doing much with remedies in your illness, or of doing nothing at all, and allowing nature to operate, which cures maladies, as our Hippocrates bears witness, you could not have applied to a person who enters more willingly into your design, and would be more prompt than I am to praise the patience and courage that you exhibit in this firm resolution. If you are of a mind to try several remedies for your relief, I feel myself capable, please God, to point out to you a great number of them, having a few good authors on the subject, which I have read and consult daily. If you or your friends have any remedies which I do not know about yet, and which are to your liking, I will not oppose your procuring them, and I will even try to find reasons, experiences, and authorities which confirm you in the resolution you have taken to employ them; but if you challenge yourself a little on your sufficiency in these matters, and that of your friends, and if you presume to know something of my studies, my experience, and my affection, you will allow me to carry on, if you please, and I can assure you that I will proceed with as much circumspection for you as for myself. Upon which I dare hope, with God's help, for a happy outcome. It is for you, Sir, to tell me which of these three ways you wish me to employ in this conjuncture, and to order those who serve you that I be exactly obeyed.

He was not sanguine that his modest proposal would be acceptable to most physicians or patients. He believed instead that it would most likely remain a "Utopian dream."

De Sorbière's reflections are an appropriate conclusion to this brief review of the "etiquette" for conversing with patients from Hippocrates through the seventeenth century. De Sorbière offers a contrast to his predecessors who considered all patients unfit for decision making, or who believed that competing considerations such as the importance of faith and reassurance to cure, pre-

cluded such practices. He at least envisioned, however ambiva-
lently, that some patients had the capacity to listen to their doctors and, on the basis of what they heard, to make their own
choices. He appreciated, though also with great reservations,
that patients would not be harmed if they were made more aware
of medicine's imperfections. Such sentiments were quite novel in
his time, as they still are in ours.

The Age of Enlightenment

During the eighteenth century a number of physicians, influenced by the spirit of the enlightenment and its vision of universal human progress and the eventual rule of reason, contended
that the public could and should be enlightened about medical
matters. Illustrious physicians such as John Gregory and Benjamin Rush spoke eloquently to the hope that an enlightened
public would become more accepting of the practice of medicine
as they felt it should be practiced. They, however, were not advocates of patient involvement in decision making. They believed
instead that patients, once they appreciated the true nature of
medicine, its great promise to alleviate suffering, would make
common cause with their doctors and accept their doctors' authority.

In 1772, John Gregory, Professor of Medicine at the University of Edinburgh, published his book "Lectures on the Duties
and Qualifications of a Physician."[30] He made a strong case for
educating laymen about health and disease. Gregory believed
that laymen should acquire some knowledge of medicine and he
urged his brethren to educate the general public, at least its more
literate members. He argued that "surely it is not a matter of
such difficulty, for a gentleman of a liberal education to learn so
much of medicine as may enable him to understand the best
books on the subject, and to judge the merits of those physicians
to whom he commits the charge of his own health, and the health
of those more immediately under his care and protection." In a
stirring concluding paragraph, he contended that the dignity of
the medical profession is not

> supported by a narrow, selfish, corporation-spirit; by self-impor-
> tance; by a formality in dress and manners, or by an affection of

mystery. The true dignity of physic is to be maintained by the superior learning and abilities of those who profess it; by the liberal manners of gentlemen; and by that openness and candour, which disdain all artifice, which invite to a free inquiry, and thus boldly bid defiance to all that illiberal ridicule and abuse, to which medicine has been so much and so long exposed.

Few listened. The traditional view that physicians must assume sole responsibility for protecting the ignorant public from its folly was too ingrained.

Yet, despite Gregory's plea for "openness and candour which disdains all artifice," his lectures remained filled with observations of traditional Hippocratic vintage that argued in favor of not taking patients into doctors' confidence. Consider, for example, his approval of the need for "an appearance of resolution, [in order not to alarm patients], even in cases where, in [the physician's own] judgment, [the doctor] is fully sensible of the difficulty." Gregory is silent on the question: When should such difficulties first be shared with patients? Or take his approval of not gratifying a patient's curiosity about the nature of the medicines prescribed for him. He based such practices on the "natural propensity in mankind to admire what is covered with the veil of obscurity, and to undervalue whatever is fully and clearly explained to them. A firm belief in the effects of a medicine depends more on the imagination, than on a rational conviction impressed on the understanding. . . ." Thus, he left us with questions: What are the limits of deception and what are the limits of decision making in physician–patient interactions when, as Gregory believed, "few people can be persuaded that a poultice of bread and milk is in many cases as efficacious as one compounded of half a dozen ingredients, to whose names they are strangers"?

Gregory did not address these and other questions because the idea of patient participation in decision making was not fully formed in his mind. It is a pity, for his commitment to equality between physicians and patients, his awareness of the treacherous pull of physicians' self-interest and caprice—and not only of patients' imbecility and caprice, as his colleague Thomas Percival would soon maintain—could have led him to make more specific recommendations that would have left an even richer and more unique legacy on the nature of physician-patient interactions. Although aware of physicians' weaknesses, patients' weaknesses loomed larger in his thinking.

Gregory perhaps saw no need to address the problem of shared decision making between physicians and patients. Raised in the Age of Enlightenment, he seemed to be convinced that reason would triumph once human beings, physicians as well as patients, were properly educated. He had high hopes for physicians:

> [A] doctor's degree can never confer sense, the title alone can never command regard. [A] physician, of a candid and liberal spirit, will never take advantage of what a nominal distinction, and certain privileges, give him over men, who, in point of real merit, are his equals; and will feel no superiority, but what arises from superior learning, superior abilities, and more liberal manners. . . .

With an abiding faith in the common sense of mankind, Gregory felt that free and informed men and women could be trusted to discover together how to live the good life. To further that objective he concentrated on those practices of his colleagues that impeded public access to knowledge about health and disease. Once that barrier had been breached, he expected physicians and patients to agree with one another since their objectives were one and the same.

His views were shared by his American contemporary, Benjamin Rush. Yet, despite some scholarly comment to the contrary,[31] neither was Rush a champion of disclosure of medical lore for purposes of gaining patients' consent. Instead, Rush expected that knowledge would set man free to act rationally. Indeed, so great was his estimate of the inherent rationality of medicine properly practiced that he believed the dissemination of medical knowledge would unite physicians and patients in a common pursuit. Now, faith in *reason*, rather than in *God* or *philia*, obviated the necessity for distinguishing between the interests of physicians and patients.

Rush urged physicians to "strip [their] profession of every thing that looks like mystery and imposture, and clothe medical knowledge in a dress so simple and intelligible, that it may become . . . obvious to the meanest capacities."[32] He asked, "shall the means . . . of preserving [health] when lost, be so abstruse, as to require years of study to discover and apply them?" And he answered his own question: "A knowledge of the virtues and doses of the most active and useful medicines, might be acquired with greater facility, and much more pleasure, than the rules for composing syllogisms laid down in our systems of logic."

While "recommending the general diffusion of medical knowledge, by making it a part of an academical education," Rush still expected properly educated patients to defer voluntarily to the authority of true medical knowledge. Until that state of grace was bestowed on mankind, Rush cautioned his colleagues to "avoid sacrificing *too much** to the taste of [their] patients. . . . Yield to them in matters of little consequence, but maintain an inflexible authority over them in matters that are essential to life." Enlightened patients, he believed, would submit to their equally enlightened physicians; for unenlightened patients, on the other hand, paternalism remained the only viable alternative.

Like Gregory, though somewhat more insistently, Rush too favored deception whenever enlightenment was not equal to the task of managing the physician-patient relationship. He was impressed by "the influence of the imagination and will upon diseases," and he admitted to having "frequently prescribed remedies of doubtful efficacy in the critical stage of acute diseases, but never till I had worked up my patients into a confidence, bordering upon certainty, of their probable good effects." Such sentiments reveal that Rush was more concerned with manipulating the physician-patient relationship for therapeutic ends than with enlightening patients to share the burdens of decision making.

Nineteenth Century Medicine

When the British and American medical associations drafted their first codes of ethics, they listened not to John Gregory's call for sharing medicine's knowledge with the public, but turned instead to Thomas Percival, a staunch advocate of good custody, even of improved custody, but not of patients' liberty. Before turning to him, I would like to stress again, lest I be misunderstood, that throughout medical history—from Hippocratic days, through the reign of Percival to the present—the physicians who wrote about medical ethics truly cared about patients' welfare. Their earnest and dedicated exhortations, admonitions, and commands were intended to improve patients' medical fate.

---

*Occasionally, to make my argument clearer, emphasis has been added in the text of a quotation, which did not appear in the original.

They were not concerned, however, with liberty, with patients' participation in decision making. The idea that such participation might be an aspect of good care had, with few exceptions, not occurred to them.

In 1791 the medical staff of the Manchester Infirmary asked the English physician Thomas Percival to draw up "a scheme of professional conduct relative to hospitals and other medical charities."[33] His colleagues hoped that such a document would settle a bitter internal dispute about professional prerogatives that had arisen among the house staff. Percival's proposals did more than that. An expanded version profoundly influenced the subsequent codification of medical ethics, particularly in the United States of America. Percival's 1803 book, *Medical Ethics: A Code of Institutes and Precepts Adapted to the Professional Conduct of Physicians and Surgeons*, served forty-four years later as the basic text for the first code of ethics of the American Medical Association.

Medical Ethics set forth principles of broad ethical significance to society and humanity as well as rules of etiquette seeking to regulate the day-to-day interactions of physicians—in hospitals and private practice—with one another as well as with apothecaries, lawyers, and judges. The principles and rules also addressed the care of patients. Percival urged his colleagues to be solicitous of their patients' welfare and to provide good custody: "Every case, committed to the charge of a physician or surgeon, should be treated with attention, steadiness and humanity."[34] The patient's right to liberty of choice, however, received no attention. For example, he admonished colleagues to heed a patient's "extreme *timidity*, with respect to venaesection," and to desist from undertaking such a procedure, if vehemently opposed. He made these recommendations not out of respect for liberty, but for their medical "[contraindications] in certain cases and constitutions." He also counseled that the "*prejudices* of the sick are not to be condemned or opposed with harshness," but not because consent deserved respect. Instead, he based his argument on therapeutic considerations, observing that even though contrariness can be "silenced by authority," such professional behavior may create "fear, anxiety and watchfulness," all detriments to patients' recovery.

Percival's brief comments on physician-patient communication focused on the limited question of whether, and to what extent, doctors should tell the truth to patients in situations of impending death. Percival followed tradition by urging restraint in making "gloomy prognostications," except "on proper occasions [when a physician should] give to the friends of the patient, timely notice of danger . . . and *even* to the patient himself, if *absolutely* necessary." And if, perchance, in suggesting that physicians say this much he had gone too far and had imposed too intolerable a burden on his colleagues, he immediately added:

> This office, however, is so peculiarly alarming, when executed by him, that it ought to be declined, whenever it can be assigned to any other person of sufficient judgment and delicacy. For the physician should be the minister of hope and comfort to the sick; that by such cordials to the drooping spirit, he may smooth the bed of death, revive expiring life, and counteract the depressing influence of those maladies which rob the philosopher of fortitude, and the Christian of consolation.

Percival seemed oblivious to the hopeless charade he had perpetrated. How could physicians, after having asked "others" to inform patients of impending death, expect "to be ministers of hope [and to] revive expiring life," without hopelessly confusing their patients at the same time? In any case, the retreat from conversation was total.

The controversy over truthfulness about dire prognosis has divided the medical profession for centuries, with the majority of physicians consistently arguing against disclosure. The fact that some doctors have pleaded for disclosure of dire prognosis has been taken as proof of the existence of a longstanding, albeit comparatively rare, commitment to what is now called informed consent.[35] Such contentions attempt to prove too much, for none of the celebrated proponents of truthfulness based their arguments on a felt need that patients should understand their situation so that they could participate in medical decision making. Other considerations influenced the call for truthfulness.

Percival is an example in point. Years later after *Medical Ethics* was published, he apparently became troubled enough by the disparate obligations of veracity, on the one hand, and the professional duty "to be ministers of hope," on the other, that he took up the subject once again. First he reviewed the writings of the authorities on truthtelling, most of whom shared the opinion of Dr. Francis Hutcheson of Glasgow that "[n]o man censures a

physician for deceiving a patient too much dejected, by expressing good hopes of him; or by denying that he gives him a proper
medicine which he is foolishly prejudiced against: the patient af-
terwards will not reproach him for it,''[36] Percival set forth his
personal views on the question: should the obligation of physicians as "ministers of hope and comfort" be circumscribed
by adding the qualification "as far as truth and sincerity will
admit"?

"Common principles of humanity," he observed, require
practitioners to "sacrifice that delicate sense of veracity" whenever truthfulness "would be deeply injurious to" a patient. He
expected such situations to arise rarely, and thus he exhorted his
colleagues "to guard [the mind] sedulously against the injury
it may sustain by such violations of the native love of truth . . .
which is so ornamental to, and indeed forms a characteristic ex-
cellence of the virtuous man." Reading Percival in context
makes it clear that his appeal to truthfulness was grounded primarily in concerns over how lying, so at odds with *"gentlemanly"*
behavior, would affect "the sincerity, the purity, and the probity
of the physician himself." However important an insight in its
own right, it says nothing about the significance of truthfulness
for patient decision making. Indeed Percival's advice that others
be assigned the "alarming" task of truthtelling suggests an intuitive awareness that communicating the truth is more the physician's than the patient's problem.

A personal experience illustrates the persistence of this problem to the present. Some years ago, an old Jewish patriarch-phy-
sician sat next to me at Hadassah Hospital in Jerusalem. For
about an hour I had been engaged with other physicians in a
heated debate over the question of whether to disclose to patients
their hopeless prognoses. All the doctors who spoke up asserted
that patients, particularly Jewish ones, could not tolerate an
awareness of impending death. Late in the discussion, the patri-
arch leaned over and whispered into my ear, "It is not the patient who cannot tolerate hearing the truth. I could not tolerate
telling my patients the truth." His remark highlights both the
readiness of many physicians to attribute their own concerns to
patients and physicians' need not to talk about painful truths or
to speak of them only in whispers to colleagues.

Percival's commentary on truthfulness in physician-patient
communications was informed not by a concern over patients'

liberty but by abiding concern, too narrowly conceived, over providing good physical custody. Percival did not appreciate that truthfulness, liberty and good physical custody may be interrelated; Tolstoy did. In *The Death of Ivan Ilych* he described beautifully how lying interferes not only with good physical custody but also with the liberty of asking for the things that during Ivan's final days mattered most to him:

> What tormented Ivan Ilych most was the deception, that lie, which for some reason they all accepted, that he was not dying but was simply ill. . . .
>
> Apart from this lying, or because of it, what most tormented Ivan Ilych was that no one pitied him as he wished to be pitied. At certain moments after prolonged suffering he wished most of all (though he would have been ashamed to confess it) for someone to pity him as a sick child is pitied. He longed to be petted and comforted. . . . [37]

The drafters of the American Medical Association's first code of ethics followed Percival in remaining oblivious to the issue of liberty. They advanced additional reasons why liberty had to bow to custody. After reproducing all of Percival's instructions on "gloomy prognostications," they added their own postscript:

> The life of a sick person can be shortened not only by the acts, but also by the words or the manner of a physician. It is, therefore, a sacred duty to guard himself carefully in this respect, and to avoid all things which have a tendency to discourage the patient and to depress his spirits. [38]

They did not ask the question: If remaining life can be shortened and made insufferable by words, can it not just as easily be shortened and made insufferable by silence?

Neither Percival nor the drafters of the AMA Code were prepared to address these questions because they remained committed to the idea that physicians must make decisions for, and not with, patients. Percival's *Medical Ethics* was addressed to "gentlemen-physicians." Indeed he used the words "gentleman" and "physician" interchangeably. Patients, on the other hand, whenever not called patients, were elevated only to the level of "fellow creatures," a small but telling example of the inequality that governed physician-patient interactions.

Similar paternalistic sentiments pervaded the first code of the

American Medical Association which embraced Percival's views and preserved his language to a considerable extent.[39] The Code, adopted in 1847, was long, consisting of approximately 5600 words. Its "Articles," particularly on physician-patient relations, deserve careful reading (see Appendix A). They give a vivid and unselfconscious picture of the medical profession's views of its practitioners and its patients, views that have remained essentially unchanged from Hippocratic days to at least the early twentieth century, if not the present.

Like Percival, the drafters of the 1847 Code could not entertain the idea of mutual decision making between physicians and patients, for the perceived differences between the two parties were just too great. For example, the opening Article states that "[physicians] should unite tenderness with firmness, and condescension with authority, [so] as to inspire the minds of their patients with gratitude, respect and confidence." Sentiments of caring custody are conveyed in the appeal to tenderness, but the call for condescension and authority create an inhospitable climate for promoting patients' liberty. The lonely view of a doctor's world in which "there is no tribunal other than his own conscience," further precluded any role for patients' participation. The gulf was just too wide between physicians who were "required to make so many sacrifices of comfort, ease, and health" and patients, who were endowed with "mental imbecility" and "crude opinions."

The drafters, who had both inherited and accepted the gulf, bridged it with firm, condescending, and authoritarian instructions: Doctors "have a right to expect and require, that their patients should entertain a just sense of the duties which they owe to their medical attendants." As for patients, their "obedience . . . should be prompt and implicit"; they "should never converse on the subject of [their] disease" when a physician is not in attendance; nor should they "send for a consulting physician without the express consent of [the] medical attendant." Finally, patients "should always be in readiness to receive the visits of their physician, as the detention of a *few* minutes is often of *serious* inconvenience to him." Particularly striking are the provisions on consultations with other physicians. In instances of "irreconcilable diversity of opinion," the drafters recommended that "the opinion of the majority [be] decisive," with "mutual concessions." Sharing of consultants' differences of opinions with patients was not advised except under the most extreme circumstances. These provisions were eventually eliminated but in this instance they were replaced by the following paragraph which only partially re-dressed the problem of secrecy:

> Should the attending physician and the consultant find it impos-sible to agree in their view of a case another consultant should be called . . . or the first consultant should withdraw. However, since the consultant was employed by the patient [to obtain] his opinion, *he should be permitted* to state [it] to the patient, his next friend in the presence of the physician in charge.[40]

The 1847 Code, promulgated by members of an association that would soon dominate American medicine, should not be dis-missed as a historic relic. It remains unique in two ways: being of relatively recent vintage, it gives a remarkably clear picture of physicians' perceptions of patients; although the Articles pertain-ing to the duties of physicians to their patients were eliminated in 1903, they were not replaced by new Articles on the subject. In-deed, beginning with the Code's first revision in 1903, and con-tinuing in the 1912, 1957, and 1980 revisions, Articles that ap-parently proved troublesome were subjected to wholesale deletions rather than to careful modification. Thus, the approxi-mately 5600 words of the 1847 Code were reduced to 4000 by 1903, 3000 by 1912, 500 by 1957, and to 250 words by 1980. To be sure, the last two versions were augmented by the Opinions of the AMA's Judicial Council that interpreted the *Principles* (as the *Code* is now called). These Opinions, however, had relatively lit-tle to say on physician-patient relations and what they did say on that subject addressed by and large special and limited groups of patients and not the vast number of patients whom physicians encounter in their practice. The original sentiments, so it seems, lived on in spirit, although not in the printed words, for physi-cians were not given new and reasonably specific instructions on how to interact with patients.

The penultimate *Principles* of 1957 compressed all prior prin-ciples on physician-patient relations into one sentence: "The prime objective of the medical profession is to render service to humanity with full respect for both the dignity of man and the rights of patients."[41] Neither the *Principles* nor the *Opinions of the AMA's Judicial Council* which interpreted the *Principles*, clarified what such respect required of physicians in their interactions with patients. The 1957 *Opinions* only provided three specific instructions with respect to disclosure and consent: (1) that a surgeon is obligated to disclose "all facts relevant to the need and the performance of the operation"; (2) that an experimenter is obligated, when using new drugs and procedures, to obtain "the voluntary consent of the person"; and (3) that investigators engaged in clinical-investigations-primarily-for-treatment must "make relevant disclosure and obtain the voluntary consent of patients or their legally authorized representative."[42] The first provision was added to comply with malpractice law, and the other two to comply with congressional legislation on the conduct of research.

The 1980 *Principles of Medical Ethics* (see Appendix B), said little about physician-patient relations: A physician shall "respect . . . human dignity" (Principle I), and "respect the rights of patients" (Principle IV). The *Current Opinions of the Judicial Council* promulgated in 1981 to accompany the 1980 Principles, however, finally addressed the issue of informed consent.[43] In paragraph 8.07 the Council stated that:

> [t]he patient's right of self-decision can be effectively exercised only if the patient possesses enough information to enable an intelligent choice. The patient should make his own determination on treatment. Informed consent is a basic social policy for which exceptions are permitted (1) where the patient is unconscious or otherwise incapable of consenting and harm from failure to treat is imminent; or (2) when risk-disclosure poses such a serious psychological threat of detriment to the patient as to be medically contraindicated. Social policy does not accept the paternalistic view that the physician may remain silent because divulgence might prompt the patient to forego needed therapy. Rational, informed patients should not be expected to act uniformly, even under similar circumstances, in agreeing to or refusing treatment.

Several things stand out. Most obvious is the Council's acknowledgment that this requirement is based on "*social* policy" generated by forces outside the medical profession. Second, physicians are provided with no information or guidance as to what "social policy" requires them to disclose so that patients can give an informed consent. For example, how much information is enough "to enable an intelligent choice"? What constitutes an "intelligent choice," particularly since law only requires a "reasonable'' choice? The Council must have known that answers to such questions are not self-evident. Moreover, only four paragraphs later, in a brief section on ''Patient Information,'' the Council retreated from its endorsement of the doctrine of informed consent by reminding physicians that they must only ''properly inform the patient of the nature and purpose of the treatment undertaken or prescribed.'' It is precisely this ancient minimal disclosure requirement that judges had found wanting and had tried to expand through their informed consent doctrine.

Most striking is the contrast between the absence of any specific advice on how to implement the informed consent obligation and the much more explicit, detailed advice proferred by the Council with respect to less significant and rarer medical situations. For example, in Paragraph 2.03, the Council advised that, in instances of artificial insemination, the consent of both the woman and her husband be obtained and that they be told that any resulting child ''is possessed of and entitled to all the rights of a child conceived naturally.'' In the following paragraph, which deals with in vitro fertilization, the Council opined that women should give their consent in writing and should be fully apprised of ''[a]lternative treatment or methods of care.'' Similar suggestions are made in Paragraph 2.08, which deals with genetic engineering.

More explicit guidelines were also given for disclosures necessary to obtain informed consent in clinical investigations (¶2.05). And, Paragraph 2.09(4), which deals with organ transplants, advises physicians to

> be objective in discussing the procedure, in disclosing known risks and possible hazards, and in advising of the alternative procedures available. The physician should not encourage expectations beyond those which the circumstances justify. The physician's interest in advancing scientific knowledge must always be secondary to his primary concern for the patient.

Why was the approach to informed consent so piecemeal? Why did it ignore both the most common and the most critical medical situations where the issue of informed consent arises? The preceding review of the AMA *Principles* and *Opinions* can lead to only one conclusion: that, for therapeutic settings, the medical profession has at best taken a first and most tentative step toward promulgating an authoritative position on disclosure and consent.

Twentieth Century Medicine

Before extending my observations on the status of disclosure and consent in this century beyond my discussion of the AMA *Principles*, I would like to add to prior comments on the relationship between truthtelling and physician-patient decision making. Richard C. Cabot, whom Paul White, his equally illustrious Harvard colleague, had called one of those "restless souls who cannot be made to fit the common mold,"[44] is best remembered as the father of the Clinicopathological Conference which, following its birth at the Massachusetts General Hospital in 1910, was quickly adopted by most teaching hospitals throughout the United States. He is less remembered for his magnificent essay on "The Use of Truth and Falsehood in Medicine: An Experimental Study," published in 1909.[45] This passionate and relentless indictment of the use of falsehood in physician-patient interactions is unparalleled in the medical literature. Cabot's total disdain for deception constituted a radical break with the more qualified views on truthtelling such as those of Gregory, Rush, and Percival. Cabot's views have at times been misinterpreted as evidence of his commitment to what is now called informed consent.

Cabot was concerned about other consequences of lying:

> We think we can isolate a lie as we do a case of smallpox, and let its effect die with the occasion that brought it about. But is it not common experience that such customs are infectious and spread far beyond our intention and beyond our control? They beget, as a rule, not any acute indignation among those who get wind of them (for 'how,' they say, 'could the doctor do otherwise'), but rather a quiet, chronic incredulity which is stubborn. . . .

He believed that lying undermines trust, if not the patient's then surely that of future patients. He admitted that lies may save a patient

> some suffering. But consider a minute. His wife has now acquired, if she did not have it already, a knowledge of the circumstances under which doctors think it merciful and useful to lie. She will be sick

herself some day, and when the doctors tell her that she is not seriously ill, is she likely to believe them?

Cabot believed that a more honest relationship between physicians and patients would reinforce patients' confidence and the authority of the physician. The importance he assigned to trust was based on his conviction that good medical custody required it, and not that patient liberty dictated it. Nowhere in his book, or in other writings that I have consulted, did Cabot address the issue of patients' rights and needs to participate in decision making. There is no reason to assume that Cabot's thoughts on the issue of doctors' authority, except on the question of deception, were out of step with the mainstream of medical thinking of his day.

Cabot's great contribution to physician-patient dialogue is to be found in his unrelenting advice to his colleagues that patients can be trusted to hear medical truths. Since trust between physicians and patients is a requisite for joint decision making, he addressed one of the necessary preconditions for mutual deliberations. Cabot did not take a next step: to advocate that physicians and patients make decisions jointly.

Since the promulgation of the informed consent doctrine in 1957, physicians have of necessity become more aware of their new obligation to talk with patients about recommended treatments. Yet, by and large any disclosures have been limited to informing patients about the risks and benefits of proposed treatments, not about alternatives, and surely not about the certainties and uncertainties inherent in most treatment options. Most importantly, conversations with patients are not conducted in the spirit of inviting patients to share with their physicians the burdens of decision. Without such a commitment, dialogue is reduced to a monologue.

Thus, what passes today for disclosure and consent in physician-patient interactions is largely an unwitting attempt by physicians to shape the disclosure process so that patients will comply with their recommendations. In a recent discussion on informed consent, a group of senior surgeons seemed genuinely puzzled by the "quaint" informed consent rule, particularly since they were certain that they could always guide patients to accept the treatment they had selected for them. "Why," they asked, "should we be forced to go through a ritual that ultimately accomplishes so little?'' I responded by asking how they would react if law at some time in the future attempted through informed consent to make patients co-decision makers? They thought that such an objective would be totally unrealistic, if not dangerous. ''Patients,'' they asserted, ''do not have the capacity to make medical decisions.''

The contemporary proponents of informed consent come largely from the field of bio-ethics and most of them are non-physicians, although there are some notable exceptions. The resistance among physicians to joint decision making has not substantially diminished, and even the more limited obligations imposed by the legal doctrine have met strong opposition. Consider these recent statements by physicians: that law's disclosure obligations extend to disclosures of every minute detail ''[filling] patients with uncertainties, [torturing] them with potentialities, however remote''[46]; that informed consent endangers patients' mental and physical life[47] and ''destroys good patient care''[48]; and that ''[t]here oughta be a law against this law.''[49]

That doctors have distorted law's commands, and then attacked their own distortions, is one thing and more easily remediable than physicians' deep-seated enmity to patients' participation in decision making. A distinguished surgeon wrote:

> [T]here is no way that I can see that a patient can logically judge whether he should have a cardiac valve replacement or not, or when, or whether it is to be with the Starr valve, a Bjork-Shiley valve, a Magovern valve, a Hancock preserved porcine valve, etc. . . . The objection of some of the laymen concerned about the problem has been to what they call the ''father knows best'' authoritative, paternalistic attitude of physicians. In fact, if ''father'' didn't know best, he ought to retire from practice.[50]

Patients may not understand the technical differences between different valves, but they can understand the alternative risks and benefits of choosing one valve over another and the impact of each choice on their well-being. For example, one valve may be safer but require earlier replacement than another; a new valve may show greater promise of providing significant relief, but data on it may be less conclusive than those on older models. At the very least, is it so difficult to imagine that patients should have some say about when to have a valve replacement, for example, before or after a grandchild's wedding?

The inquiry on shared decision making is not advanced by saying, as has become recent practice, and as the surgeon went on to say at the point I interrupted his quote, "[t]his is not to say that every effort should not be made to explain in reasonable degree, and to the degree the patient wishes it explained, what is in prospect for him." As long as such sentiments stand alone, they are meaningless. At a minimum, they require some elaboration of what is meant by the phrases "to explain in reasonable degree" and "what is in prospect for him." Both sentiments can require the most extensive or most limited explanations. The absence of medical commentary on what constitutes reasonable explanations for purposes of patient consent make such elaborations essential in order to improve the climate of decision making between physicians and patients.

Summing up

The history of the physician-patient relationship from ancient times to the present bears testimony to physicians' caring dedication to their patients' physical welfare. The same history, by its account of the silence that has pervaded this relationship, also bears testimony to physicians' inattention to their patients' right and need to make their own decisions. Little appreciation of disclosure and consent can be discerned in this history, except negatively, in the emphasis on patients' incapacities to apprehend the mysteries of medicine and therefore, to share the burdens of decision with their doctors.

It is the history of silence with respect to patient participation in decision making that I wanted to document in this chapter. Challenging the long-standing tradition of silence requires nothing less than uprooting the prevailing authoritarian value and belief systems and replacing them with more egalitarian ones. If my diagnosis is correct, the remedy is barely in sight.

In the light of the history of silence it would be surprising, indeed suspect, if the recent interest in disclosure and consent had already made significant inroads on existing practices. As Freud observed, "[t]he past, the tradition of the race [to which I would add 'and of the profession'] live on in the ideologies of the super-ego, and yield only slowly to the influence of the present and to new changes."[51] The residues left behind in the conscience of the professional, informed by ancient history and modern learning, cannot be easily and quickly dissolved. Thus assertions that medicine has accepted the principles of disclosure and consent and is conducting its practices in accordance with them are, at best, suspect, and, at worst, dangerous nonsense.

Alasdair MacIntyre's recent observations on physican-patient decision making perceptively assess its current status:

> Traditionally, the patient puts himself in the doctor's hands. The doctor generally in return does not advise the patient of a variety of possibilities and leave the patient to decide; he generally does not in fact reveal to the patient his own processes of thinking. . . . In our culture only this kind of medical authority does not appear to us as odd and singular as it is, because we are familiarized with it from early childhood; but when we do learn to notice it, its oddity is all the more obtrusive because it is so very nearly without parallel in the rest of our social experience.[52]

MacIntyre, however, is mistaken in calling such medical conduct "without parallel." It is deeply embedded in the ethos of all professions. In their political struggles both to gain control over their practices through exclusive licensure laws and to secure freedom from lay control, all professions have sought to impose their authority on the public. I now turn to the history of the medical profession as a political organization and to the contribution that this history has made to the silent world of doctor and patient.

II

Physicians and Citizens: The Struggle for Freedom from Lay Control

THIS ACCOUNT OF MEDICINE'S HISTORY as a political institution is intended to demonstrate that physicians' political and social philosophy about public health only gave more far-reaching expression to what they believed to be true for the more intimate interpersonal context: that lay persons, like patients, had little to contribute to medical decision making, that fundamental inequalities between doctors and the laity created an unbridgeable chasm. Over many centuries, competing groups of healers struggled with each other and with the public for control over the nation's health care needs. The various groups had little in common except an abiding conviction that only health care providers could pass judgment on the qualities that they should possess and the kind of health care that should be available to the public. This conviction fueled the quest for political power.

While resistance to physicians' demands for obedience to their orders did not surface in the interpersonal arena of doctors' offices, it did emerge in the larger political arena. In the latter less threatening and more impersonal context, dissatisfaction with doctors' practices could more readily be expressed. For centuries, the citizens of England refused to grant any of the warring groups of healers the long-sought exclusive prerogative to control the health needs of all patients. The interprofessional struggle for supremacy that began in Europe almost a thousand years ago was finally won in the United States around the turn of this century by university-trained "regular" physicians—or allopaths, as they were called.

It was no accident that the power struggle among competing groups to obtain an exclusive mandate to practice medicine was waged through the political process rather than through individual citizens' acceptance of doctors' services. The therapeutic successes claimed by the various professional groups, as well as the therapeutic failures with which they charged one another, could not easily be supported by convincing evidence. While each group could point to singular achievements to advance its claim to pre-eminence, it was equally true that all groups had their share of inexplicable successes and failures. Each celebrated its own successes and indicted all others with their failures, but none could offer satisfactory accounts of why various remedies had succeeded or failed. Since they could not rely on reason to establish their claims, they sought to enlist the authority of the state to confirm their credentials and, in turn, to gain exclusive control.

The inability of any group to make a good case on the basis of solid evidence for being singled out as the only legitimate descendant of Aesculapias led each group to assert that the esoteric nature of its craft was understandable only to the initiated, that laymen could not distinguish between "charlatans" and true professionals. The superiority of one group over the others therefore had to be taken by the public on faith. Even non-medical healers who decried the obfuscations and the lack of common sense of university-trained practitioners made similar claims. They, too, found it difficult to explicate their practices when confronted with the successes of other healers who had employed vastly different treatments.

It is ironic that allopathic physicians, while dismissive of lay judgments, finally attained their objective by petitioning lay state officials to grant them exclusive authority. It is equally ironic that when these petitions were granted, legislators for the most part acceded to physicians' contentions that successful practice required freedom from lay control. Indeed, physicians seemed to

have it both ways. In recent decades, however, the alliance between legislatures and the medical profession that was forged
then has proven to be a mixed blessing for physicians. It has
opened the door to increased state regulation of professional
practices.

The state's selection of allopathic medicine was settled not by
reason but by faith in the prospect that its particular knowledge
would ultimately prove more beneficial to all citizens' health
needs. The possession of such esoteric knowledge, which was
only acquired after intensive study and which laypersons could
not understand, was the major justification advanced by allopaths for freedom from lay control. Public concern over exploitation and other abuses of authority was countered by physicians'
claims of altruistic and dedicated commitment to their patients'
welfare, as prescribed by their codes of ethics. Thus, they argued
that doctors deserved the unqualified trust of patients and the
public. I shall discuss the protection that altruism provides and
the problem of trust in Chapter IV. Here I would like to trace allopaths' long march from modest beginnings to pre-eminence, a
history shared with professionals in other fields. A review of the
development of professionalism in medicine may shed some light
on the political, social, and professional forces that have shaped
medicine's impact on our contemporary culture and on the lives
of patients.

The Origin of Professionalism

The historical origins of the professions, and the forces that contributed to their evolution, are shrouded in mystery. Historians
seem to agree, however, that the earliest antecedents of the professions as we know them today are to be found in eleventh century Europe. Around that time, cities increased in numbers, and
individuals engaged in common pursuits felt a need to band
together in "associations." Physicians, lawyers, merchants,
craftsmen, and even lowly water-bearers joined groups for social,
self-protective and, later, educational purposes. Teachers and
students formed associations too, and from these the universities
evolved.[1]

Uniting in associations and projecting an identifiable image
to the outside world permitted more formal and structured op-

portunities for social and professional intercourse. The initial objective of the associations was not the regulation of the practices of its own members, but rather control over the professional practices each considered to be within its province, and, in turn, the exclusion of all other groups from similar practice. The possibility of living side by side with fellow professionals of different persuasions, who belonged to their own separate associations, was rejected out of hand. Ultimately, all "deviant" professional groups had to be eliminated, even at the price of absorbing some of their members into the dominant group or of letting them quietly practice until retirement.

Close ties were soon established between universities, the Church, medicine, and law. Initially, the clergy dominated. Indeed, in those early days, only persons who had taken ecclesiastical orders were permitted to become doctors of medicine or lawyers. As the religious links loosened—gradually, at first, and, after Henry VIII came to power, at an ever accelerating pace— close ties were forged between professors, lawyers, clergy, and physicians, all of whom were university-trained.

The early and close ties among the "educated" groups created a small but powerful elite that had the ear of kings, and, later, of Parliament, city councils, and other legislative bodies. United in the common pursuit of authority and power over ordinary citizens, these groups tended to support one another, particularly in relation to the wide world of patients, clients, lay healers and lay advisors whom, like the rest of mankind, they considered uneducated and of little consequence. This history set the stage for designation of university-trained doctors of medicine as the only "true" practitioners of medicine when the public finally acquiesced to the legislative decision of selecting one group over all others.

Early Struggles among Competing Groups

Medicine struggled for a long time to reach its current status. During most of mankind's history physicians were not as powerful as they are today. Paul Starr has presented extensive evidence that well into the nineteenth century American physicians were underpaid and commanded little respect.[2]

The lack of respect by the public is reflected in the limited success of physicians' first attempts to obtain an exclusive mandate to practice. One of the earliest surviving documents reveals that in the early fourteenth century, the renowned, university-educated physician Gilbert Kymer petitioned the Mayor of London to delegate control over medical licensing and practice in the city to the professional organization to which he belonged. It is uncertain whether the petition was granted. If it was, the arrangement did not long survive. In the sixteenth century, the eminent English physician Thomas Linacre tried again. Licensing laws were passed but they applied only to physicians residing within four miles of London and their enforcement was placed under the jurisdiction of the Bishop of London and his officers, aided by four doctors of medicine. At the same time, the practice of "physic and surgery" by unlicensed practitioners (the so-called "domestic practitioners") was forbidden. The radius of the licensing authority was extended to seven miles by Henry VIII in 1518, who also went one step further by assigning to the newly chartered Royal College of Physicians the task of enforcing his orders.

The exclusivity of even such limited arrangements proved illusory. Despite all official prohibitions, unlicensed healers, such as apothecaries, barber-surgeons, wise women, ministers, farriers, and other "domestic practitioners," attended to the health needs of the public side by side with licensed university-trained "doctors of medicine." Indeed, unofficial toleration of all kinds of practitioners, was the rule from the eleventh century to the end of the nineteenth century. As one medical historian has put it, "[s]ome kind of medical treatment was available to nearly all, but all did not have to submit to the same type. The physician who arrived in sartorial splendor, waving his gold-headed cane and spouting Latin aphorisms, was likely to have the same reassuring effect on a gentleman that an experienced village woman would have on her neighbor."[3]

Many of the domestic practitioners were renowned in their communities for their medical skills and had a large following. Among them were healers who possessed remarkable intuition and had acquired a considerable amount of medical lore. They knew how to administer medicinal plants in homeopathic doses. They possessed the wisdom to practice judiciously, largely limiting their interventions to lending nature a helping and comforting hand. Although not professionally trained in any formal sense, they must be distinguished from "quacks," particularly the group of peripatetic mountebanks who became notorious during American Colonial days for setting up stages, selling nostrums to the accompaniment of theatrical entertainment, and then fleeing, often never to return.

To be sure, domestic practitioners had their share of ignorant and incompetent pretenders as did doctors of medicine. Until the twentieth century, standards of medical training varied greatly. For centuries, a university medical degree could be obtained almost for the asking. As President Eliot of Harvard observed, even in the late nineteenth century, anybody could "walk into a medical school from the street," and many who did walk in "could barely read and write."[4] It was only in 1910 that Columbia University required entering medical students to be high school graduates.

Since the public could not distinguish between the qualified and unqualified on the basis of formal training, patients wisely preferred to trust reputation as transmitted by word of mouth. As a result, the general public frequently placed greater faith in domestic practitioners than in university-educated physicians, so that the learned professions' efforts to bar unlicensed persons from the practice of medicine by exclusive licensing laws were for a long time doomed to failure.

These patterns of English medical practice were brought to Colonial America. Domestic practitioners practiced side by side with the handful of university-trained doctors who had emigrated to the New World. The distinctions between "regular" and "empirical" (domestic) practitioners remained blurred. The latter were not deterred from practicing; constraints were limited to occasional legislation that imposed the ineffectual penalty of prohibiting unlicensed healers from suing for nonpayment of fee. These counterproductive laws permitted domestic practitioners to ask in good conscience for payment prior to treatment. In the heady expectation of cure, patients complied willingly. If anyone was penalized by such legislation, it was the regular practitioner.

During Colonial and early post-revolutionary days, American legislators and judges were generally quite tolerant of diverse and competing medical groups. They tried to protect the public not by adjudicating which group was the most competent but by making sure, as best they could, that members of each group had acquired the highest level of competence established by their respective group of practitioners. For example, an early Massachusetts statute required that persons be skilled in the "approved Rules of Art, in each Mystery and occupation" and seek "the advice and consent of such as are skillful in the same Art, (if such may be had) or at least some of the wisest and gravest then present."[5] Or, as an early Iowa judge observed with respect to the question of adjudicating the competence of competing groups:

> It is to be lamented, that so many of our citizens are disposed to trust, health and life to novices and empirics, to new nostrums and new methods of treatment. But these are evils which courts of justice possess no adequate power to remedy. Enlightened public opinion, and judicious legislation, may do much to discountenance quackery, and advance medical science.[6]

The Iowa court insisted only that the physician, in this instance a botanic practitioner, possess and properly employ the ordinary skills of his group and that his patient know whom he had consulted. If injury then resulted, the patient "could properly blame no one but himself." Thus both legislation and judicial opinion stressed competence to practice one's chosen calling and citizen-patients' freedom to select from a varied menu of practitioners.

At the same time, as the Iowa opinion suggests, many judges of the last half of the nineteenth century deplored the ways in which citizens exercised their liberty. They asked for both "enlightened public opinion" and "judicious legislation" to remedy the situation, and before too long legislation was enacted that for the first time in history delegated to allopaths a virtual monopoly over medical practices. Courts upheld these laws despite many constitutional challenges. They held that states, in the exercise of their "police power," had the authority to pass laws designed "[to protect] the lives, limbs, health, comfort and convenience, as well as the prosperity, of all persons within the State."[7]

Allopaths had to mount two concerted efforts before American legislators were finally persuaded to grant them a virtual monopoly over American medical practice. The first effort, during the early nineteenth century, assigned licensing authority largely to incorporated medical societies. By 1830, 13 states had passed such laws. Yet, within two decades, all such laws were repealed and the first American legislative attempt to distinguish between "trained" and "empirical" practitioners ended in failure.

Pioneer America distrusted specialists. Its confidence in common sense of citizens extended to the management of illness, which it believed should be left to citizens' individual judgment. The idea of a profession with special prerogatives was repugnant to a rising American democracy. To prescribe high qualifications for, and to limit access to, a profession seemed undemocratic and un-American. Moreover, domestic practice and folk medicine were still firmly entrenched, and when their adherents rallied and petitioned their legislators, they routed the opposition.

Thomsonians, Homeopaths, and Allopaths

The history of medical licensure differed somewhat from state to state, with the northeastern experience, leading up to the second wave of exclusive licensure laws, ultimately shaping the future of American medicine in decisive ways. While in early nineteenth century New England and other northeastern states a wide variety of healers practiced side by side, three major groups began to dominate the medical scene: among domestic practitioners, the Thomsonians, and among university-trained physicians, the more recent homeopaths and the older and more numerous allopaths.

Samuel Thomson, a New Hampshire farmer who founded the Thomsonian sect, developed a system of therapy based on the curative effects of a few herbal stimulants, emetics, and the application of heat. He and his disciples practiced full-time, published journals, and established professional societies, but they did not create any formal educational institutions. Thomsonians insisted that their therapy was not merely an alternative to orthodox medicine but that it alone was based on tried and true medical principles. They railed against the unnecessary obscurity of medicine. Physicians, said Thomson, "have learned just enough to know how to deceive people, and keep them in ignorance, by covering their doings under a language unknown to their patients."[8] The fact that some of Thomson's followers sought to establish a medical school and impose restrictions on practice, which Thomson opposed, underscores the powerful need for privilege and status even among those with an avowed faith in the simplicity and easy accessibility of medical knowledge.

Thomson's cause quickly evolved into a crusade. During the

1830's and '40s Thomsonians enjoyed a considerable public following. For example, in New York they secured legislative repeal of all penalties that had been levelled against unlicensed practitioners, including the prohibition against suing for fees. After a few decades, however, Thomsonianism went into a rapid decline for reasons that are not entirely clear. A contributing factor probably was the increasing value the public placed on higher education.

The victory of allopaths over homeopaths is ironic in the history of professional dominance. While both were university-trained, many homeopathic physicians were distinguished graduates of European medical schools, and thus were better educated than most of the allopaths. Therefore, allopathic practitioners could not charge homeopaths with a lack of formal education as they had done with the Thomsonians. Moreover, the homeopaths were also the more "scientific" practitioners. They were firmly committed to a theory of therapeutics, albeit one that was eventually discredited, which stated that diseases could be cured by administering minute doses of remedies that produced symptoms similar to those of the disease for which they were prescribed. They also took an interest in clinical investigations by testing their remedies on human subjects. Theory and experimental clinical trials, not empiricism—a practice based on clinical experience without the aid of a theory and science—guided their therapeutic practices.

The allopaths employed two techniques to defeat the homeopaths. First, they established an ever increasing number of medical schools, thereby maintaining numerical superiority over their rivals. That strategy not only gave them great political influence, but also made them more visible to the public. At the same time, the uncontrolled proliferation of allopathic medical schools produced physicians who were marginally trained at best. Second, in response to the homeopaths' dogmatic but "scientific" theories on the nature of disease, the allopaths espoused a great commitment to free and open inquiry and to the value of observation and eclecticism. The disdain of cold theory and the avowal of clinical experience that seemed more responsive to patients' individual needs and that was so similar to the approach of domestic practitioners, made allopaths more appealing to the public who had for generations relied on unlicensed healers.

For a while, perhaps also out of a sense of affinity for other university-trained practitioners, many allopathic medical societies permitted homeopaths to participate in their activities as full members. Homeopaths were also considered regular practitioners under the laws of some states. Yet, as allopaths and homeopaths practiced side by side, homeopaths gradually became more popular because they shared one characteristic with domestic practitioners that patients appreciated. Homeopaths prescribed minute doses of drugs that avoided the deleterious side-effects of allopaths' more powerful pharmacological prescriptions. Patients found such prescriptions, like the herbal medicines of many domestic practitioners, more to their taste. Homeopaths' popularity soon aggravated the latent and unavoidable power struggle between the two competing professional groups and around the turn of this century, after many professional and legislative battles, allopathy emerged victorious.

Medical Monopoly and the Age of Science

The final defeat of all their competitors gave allopaths a virtual monopoly over American medical practices. Once their legislative mandates had been secured allopaths could begin the internal rebuilding of medicine in earnest. They could raise standards of admission and training without fear of losing prospective students to other groups. They no longer had to accommodate lay groups for political considerations, or special favors and privileges beyond those of other healers. Both medicine and patients benefitted from the resulting improvements in the technical competence of physicians.

Yet the achievement of a substantial monopoly also allowed the medical profession to exert greater control over everything that impinged on its sense of mission. In particular, the allopaths' monopoly reinforced the historical belief that physicians, and not patients, should control all aspects of medical practice. Since they no longer had to defend themselves against the criticism of rival groups, doctors asserted more adamantly, and now without fear of contradiction, that laymen could not judge medical practices and had to comply with medical orders. Since patients had nowhere else to turn, it is not surprising that medical educators, while improving the technical competence of physicians, saw no need to upgrade the embryonic state of patients' participation in decision making.

While these legislative battles were being fought, a revolutionary development was taking place within medicine itself. A small number of academic physicians and non-medical scientific investigators were beginning to make remarkable discoveries that would soon capture the public imagination. They developed a vaccine against rabies, a most feared disease; they established the bacterial etiology of many diseases that led to expectations of finding cures for equally dreaded diseases, such as tuberculosis and the plague; they recognized the importance of surgical asepsis and discovered the anesthetic value of ether that would soon allow surgeons to cure diseases hitherto beyond the reach of their scalpels.

The age of science in medicine—the radical transformation of medicine that began in mid-nineteenth century and continues today—coincided with the age of medical monopoly. While scientific thinking in medicine existed at least as early as the seventeenth century, the decisive change in the mid-nineteenth century was the startling rapidity of medical advances which profoundly changed the profession. It is this transformation of medicine during the last 150 years that I want to capture under the phrase "the age of science." The magical promise of science to wipe out disease contributed to the public's willingness to turn away from other healers and allow allopaths, whose handful of scientific brethren had been associated with these discoveries, to take charge of the nation's health needs.

Yet, at first, the majority of allopathic physicians took little interest in these new developments. While they were quite willing to incorporate any scientific discoveries of therapeutic value into their practices they did not then, and even now, seriously confront the question of whether the advent of science necessitated a radical break with two millenia of Hippocratic medical practices based on clinical judgment and experience alone.

Medicine's widely publicized scientific discoveries endeared allopathic physicians to the public. Allopaths began to capitalize on these sentiments in order to consolidate the legal power that the legislative mandate to control medical practices had given them. Increasingly they emphasized a commitment to a practice of medicine based on scientific principles. The American Medical Association expressed its commitment indirectly in the 1912 revision of the *Principles* by urging its members to join medical societies in order "[to promote] the advancement of medical science."[9]

The history of allopathy, however, made it difficult for such a commitment to be more than an aspiration for practicing physicians, at least for a long time to come. Indeed, the discrepancy between aspiration and reality created tensions that continue to plague medical practices. While the small number of physicians who contributed to medicine's scientific revolution came largely from the ranks of allopaths, the majority of allopathic physicians, except for possessing an M.D. degree, had less in common with these scientist-physicians and more with the domestic practitioners. Indeed, it must be remembered that the allopaths' victory over the homeopaths had been due in part to their avowed eclecticism and emphasis on observation and clinical experience rather than dogma, be it scientific or otherwise. In these respects allopaths were quite similar to domestic practitioners. At the same time scientific developments also began to capture the public imagination and to stimulate a heady faith in the curative potential of scientific medicine. This paradox may reflect a public yearning for both the personal care associated with the domestic practitioners and the new magical cures of scientific medicine.

The disparate objectives of allopathic medicine created confusion among the ranks of its practitioners. Allopaths achieved their power both by publicly espousing values that actually went contrary to the ethos of science and by formally embracing values that as official policy promoted science. The controversy within the profession over the respective virtues of a practice based on scientific evidence versus one based on clinical experience continues to this day and results from modern medicine's mixed origins.

Allopathy has never represented a homogeneous group of practitioners or points of view with respect to theory and practice. Yet the establishment of a medical monopoly, which quite naturally tended to emphasize commonality of practice rather than diversity, has beclouded the fact that the M.D. degree does not suggest that those who possess it necessarily espouse similar treatment philosophies. The focus here is not on differences in competence among individual practitioners or in treatment philosophies among subspecialists and the problems such differences can create for patients whenever they consult first, and for the same condition, a surgeon, internist, or psychiatrist; instead, the focus is on the sharp cleavages between allopaths committed to the practice of scientific medicine and those for whom clinical experience and judgment are everything. This unacknowledged tension between the contemporary official dogma of a practice based on scientific principles and the contrary reality has confused and disoriented patients to a greater extent than has commonly been appreciated.

It may not be far-fetched to suggest that the much lamented modern demand for non-M.D. healers, even faith healers, is influenced by this disorientation. For example, some patients find it difficult to distinguish between the less scientifically minded M.D. physicians they have encountered and the physician-dispensers of laetrile who are the modern descendants of domestic practitioners. With doctors who have little commitment to the ethos of science continuing to exert a considerable influence over medical practice, the centuries-old struggle between university-trained and domestic practitioners is covertly maintained, albeit now with both being part of the same professional group.

Alvan R. Feinstein has aptly described the contemporary status of the scientific practice of medicine:

> Neither the Hippocratic Oath nor any of the modern codes of medical ethics [provide] an assurance about what is probably the most important assumption that a patient makes in seeking medical care . . . that the doctor's good intentions are accompanied by a scientific knowledge. . . .
>
> . . . The pledges contain no statements about seeking and getting scientific evidence to prove the value of medical treatments. Nor is there any pledge of using scientific methods in the doctor's challenge of evaluating risk-benefit ratios, designing reproducible successes, and avoiding self-delusion in contemplating the results.
>
> . . . The best a patient can hope for is that the doctor will be tested and certified to carry out whatever wisdom (or folly) constitutes the accepted therapeutic standards of the era.[10]

Feinstein is correct. Neither codes of medical ethics nor licensing laws provide an assurance to patients that the allopathic physicians they consult adhere to reasonably similar treatment philosophies.

Modern Medicine: An Amalgam of Science and Intuition

The modern evolution of the medical profession was decisively affected by allopaths' diversity at a crucial moment in history. The simultaneous occurrence of two revolutionary events—a political one, the imminent opportunity to obtain an exclusive legislative mandate over the practice of medicine, and a medical one, the imminent possibility of attaining pre-eminence as a result of the scientific transformation of medicine—raises an intriguing question: why did allopaths persist in enlisting the authority of the state at a time when medicine was making such spectacular advances that its pre-eminence among competing groups appeared within reach on those grounds alone? Why did they seek lay legislative assistance to gain supremacy when it would only create new problems? Why did they not let the marketplace prevail in the expectation that scientific medicine would soon vanquish all competing groups by the sheer weight of its successes?

Many reasons can be offered for the choice of a legislative resolution. Some that have frequently been identified are: (1) the well-nigh irresistible impulse, in the light of the historically bitter struggles between competing groups of healers, to strike while the iron was hot and to fulfill the ancient dreams of Gilbert Kymer, Thomas Linacre and countless other university-trained physicians to control apprenticeship and licensing; (2) physicians' hope that an exclusive mandate to practice would permit them to channel the energy they previously had expended in fighting competing groups and currying public favor into raising standards of medical school admission and training; (3) physicians' expectation that monopolistic control would allow them to restrict entry into the profession which, in turn, would improve their precarious economic status; (4) the gradual erosion of the egalitarian spirit of the Jacksonian era and its replacement by "the culture of professionalism,"[11] as Burton J. Bledstein has called it. Ambitious young men and women of the American middle class increasingly hungered for special recognition of their talents and felt professional status would distinguish them from the common people. Acquisition of professional titles became the new American dream and, in the late nineteenth century, the number of professionals began to skyrocket. These new professionals sought to protect their newly won prestige and privileges by petitioning legislatures for exclusive jurisdiction over admission and training.

Another significant reason, however, for the impetus of seeking a legislative resolution was the difficulty all healing groups experienced in giving a reasonably adequate account of their own successes and failures and, even more importantly, of competing groups' successes. Since none of them were able to establish their pre-eminence conclusively by the weight of their own activities, that distinction had to be conferred by an outside authority, the state.

With the emergence of medical science, however, allopaths might have paused, taken stock, and established a new practice of medicine based on scientific principles alone. They might have decided to treat only those patients whom they could treat by their science and leave the rest to other healers. Or, as an alternative, allopaths might have decided to stick to their self-imposed mission of being healers for all the ills of mankind, yet with greater awareness as to whom among their patients they were treating according to principles of science and whom they were not.

This did not happen and the practice of allopathic medicine continued to rest with one foot in medical science and whatever practical knowledge it provides, and the other foot in the "wisdom" of clinical experience, which is difficult to explicate and has to be taken on faith. The continuing reliance on empiricism, however, had to perpetuate the ancient struggle with pretenders. Even stringent licensing laws, as the laetrile experience illustrates, could not prevent the occasional emergence of pretenders who claimed that their clinical intuition was not different from the intuition of regular practitioners. Thus the unlicensed and the "quacks" have remained an ever-present threat to allopaths. Medical science might eventually have vanquished them but a practice based on clinical wisdom could not.

Allopaths' achievement of political supremacy, I believe, impeded the transformation of medicine in the wake of its scientific revolution which could have led to the establishment of a radically different type of practice from that known prior to the nineteenth century. Political victory allowed allopaths to rest content with having vanquished all other competing groups. Since they did not wish to undermine their newly won power in the eyes of the public by internal strife over who among them were the "true" practitioners of medicine, differences were compromised rather than resolved.

Moreover, a more complete departure from empiricism and an acceptance of science would have created new problems for allopaths. Their ability to discriminate better between knowledge and ignorance would have raised the question: Should knowledge and ignorance be shared with patients? Allopaths were unwilling and ill-prepared to address this question. Recall the inordinate importance that physicians traditionally have assigned to faith, trust, and obedience as preconditions for cure. Cure, doctors believed, required professing certainty to patients. Moreover, conversing with patients about such matters not only would have required learning a new language—how to communicate in new and unaccustomed ways—but also would have changed fundamentally the unequal relations between physicians and patients. Such revolutionary consequences were hard to contemplate. It seemed far better to maintain time-honored beliefs that patients did not have the capacity to participate in decision making and, in any case, that such invitations did not serve patients' medical interests.

A commitment to the ethos of science would have drawn attention to the tensions between ancient professional beliefs and non-disclosure, on the one hand, and science's commitment to truth and free access to information, on the other. These tensions were quickly obscured, however, by physicians' emphasis on the complexities of medical science and the limits of lay competence to grasp them. Thus, the old idea that esoteric medical knowledge is incomprehensible to laypersons was reinvoked in the name of science and its esoteric complexity.

It is a pity that the feared consequences of sharing uncertainties with patients contributed to the blurring of the boundaries of medical knowledge based on science or intuition. If physicians had increasingly spoken with patients about uncertainties, patients might have learned to distinguish physicians from quacks, and physicians committed to the practice of scientific medicine from those who based their interventions on hunch and intuition. Patients might also have learned to discriminate between treatment recommendations that were based on tested scientific evidence and those that were beset by uncertainties or based on conjecture and clinical intuition. Patients might not have become as confused as they now are. In addition, doctors would have learned whether such disclosures actually are detrimental to patients' welfare.

History did not march along these roads. Modern medicine remains caught between science and intuition. This is not necessarily bad; indeed medicine may have to be ruled by both science and intuition for a long time to come. What is disturbing, though, is that physicians are so reluctant to acknowledge to themselves and their patients which of their opinions and recommendations are based on science and which on intuition.

The recent emergence of the doctrine of informed consent could express both an awareness by a more enlightened public that with the advent of the age of science physicians can finally communicate more meaningfully with patients and a wish to provide patients with a greater opportunity to exercise control over what happens to them. A radical change in physician-patient relations may be in the making; it could reverse the misgivings, so frequently voiced in today's world, about the awesome authority that doctors silently exercise over patients' lives. Informed consent may not be a symptom of an underlying dis-ease that has affected the public, as physicians have come to believe, but an expression of a healthy wish by the public to take greater control over its medical fate. Like "laudable pus," that doctors for centuries have taken as a sign of imminent recovery from illness, informed consent may also announce the possibility of a cure for the mutual mistrust that has stalked the physician-patient relationship for centuries.

Summing up

Physicians' quest for political power mirrors the quest for interpersonal domination of the physician-patient relationship. The public's reluctance to delegate exclusive authority to one group of healers during most of medicine's history may have been symptomatic of its misgivings over the unquestioned trust and obedience that doctors demanded from their patients. These misgivings could be voiced openly in situations when the public was not in direct contact with doctors, while in more intimate encounters patients could only express them passively and silently through noncompliance with their doctors' orders.

Allopaths' legislative victory that delegated to doctors virtually monopolistic control over the health care of citizens stifled any consideration of greater patient participation in decision making. The legal doctrine of informed consent to which I now turn is an attempt by society to redress the balance, to give patients some measure of authority over their lives as patients. The analysis of this doctrine will draw sharp distinctions between informed consent's promise to provide patients with a right to self-determination and its failure to implement such an aspiration.

III

Judges, Physicians, and Patients: The Legal Doctrine of Informed Consent

T HE HISTORY OF THE DOCTRINE of informed consent illumi-
nates the difficulties of resolving the conflicting tensions
that judges were confronted with when they attempted to
extend patients' rights to self-determination. Judges perceived
the conflict to be one between liberty and caring custody. Their
ambivalence about choosing liberty over custody is well illustrated in *Faretta v. California*,[1] an opinion that passed judgment on
whether a client could be his own lawyer. In that case, the United
States Supreme Court held that the Sixth Amendment assures a
criminal defendant the constitutional right to refuse the assistance of counsel. In his opinion for the majority, Justice Stewart
asserted "[a]nd whatever else may be said of those who wrote the
Bill of Rights, surely there can be no doubt that they understood
the inestimable worth of free choice." Justice Blackman, in dis-
sent, rebutted that "[i]f there is any truth to the old proverb, that
'one who is his own lawyer has a fool for a client,' the Court by
its opinion today now bestows a *constitutional* right on one to make
a fool of himself."

Thus, it is not surprising that in the more unfamiliar settings

48

of medicine, judges have made impassioned pleas for patient self-determination, and then have undercut them by giving physicians considerable latitude to practice according to their own lights, exhorting them only to treat each patient with the utmost care. Judges could readily advance this more limited plea because generally doctors do treat their patients with solicitude. The affirmation of physicians' commitment to patients' physical needs, however, has failed to address physicians' lack of commitment to patients' decision making needs. These tensions have led judges to fashion a doctrine of informed consent that has secured for patients the right to better custody but not to liberty—the right to choose how to be treated.

The following legal history of disclosure and consent is divided into three consecutive stages: the low status of disclosure and consent from its earliest beginnings to the mid-twentieth century; the birth and development of informed consent from 1957 through 1972; and the retreat from disclosure and consent after 1972. A handful of cases will focus the inquiry; they are typical cases and not carefully selected aberrations. Had that been my objective, I could have chosen more egregious examples.

The Low Status of Disclosure and Consent

Consent to surgical interventions is an ancient legal requirement. Under the legal rubric of battery, courts jealously guarded patients' right to know and to agree to what a surgeon intended to do to them. But this right was most narrow in scope; it was merely a right of refusal. There was no right for patients to decide, after having been properly informed, whether an intervention was agreeable to them in the light of its risks and benefits as well as available alternatives. With respect to the right to know, an eighteenth century English judge observed: "a patient should be told what is about to be done to him, that he may take courage and put himself in such a situation as to enable him to undergo the operation."[2] With respect to the right to agree, a nineteenth century American judge opined, "if she voluntarily submitted to [the] performance [of the operation] her consent will be presumed, unless she was the victim of a false and fraudulent misrepresentation."[3] A physician had to inform the patient only of the *nature* of the procedure, that is, what the doctor proposed to do and, if the patient then submitted, the doctor had obtained the patient's consent. Failure to advise a patient of this minimal information and failure to respect a patient's refusal admitted of no excuse, except in an emergency or when the patient was deemed incompetent.

The two most famous and often quoted early twentieth century cases, *Pratt v. Davis* (1905)[4] and *Schloendorff v. The Society of the New York Hospital* (1914),[5] merely reaffirmed a citizen-patient's elementary right to be free from offensive (uninvited) contact. Neither Justice Brown in *Pratt* nor Justice Cardozo in *Schloendorff*, broke new legal ground. The cases did not establish a patient's right to "thoroughgoing self-determination" in medical decision making. A careful look at the facts of both cases and the judicial holdings makes it clear that patients' rights were much more narrowly conceived.

Pratt v. Davis (1905)

Mrs. Parmelia Davis, a 40-year-old housewife, had been suffering from epilepsy for many years. When her husband heard that a Dr. Pratt was considered an authority on the treatment of this condition, he arranged for his wife to see him. After his examination, Dr. Pratt concluded that to cure the epilepsy both her uterus and ovaries needed to be excised. The doctor performed this operation without informing the patient of the nature of the surgery. The doctor insisted that he had told the husband the truth, although Mr. Davis claimed otherwise, but he admitted that he had withheld this information from the patient. Since "he wished her to come to the operating room without violence,"[6] he had spoken to her only of his intention to repair a few superficial cervical and rectal tears. He told the court quite unselfconsciously that "[h]e did not deem her worthy [of any explanation];" that he had "worked her deliberately, systematically, taking chances which she did not realize the full aspect of [and that he had] deliberately and calmly deceived the woman." Through his attorney, Dr. Pratt also quite unselfconsciously advanced the proposition that "when a patient places herself in the care of a surgeon for treatment without [express limitations] upon his authority, she thereby in law consents that he may perform such operation as in his best judgment is proper and essential to her welfare.'' In inspired language the court repudiated this claim:

> [U]nder a free government at least, the free citizen's first and greatest right, which underlies all the others—the right to the inviolability of his person, in other words, his right to himself—is the subject of universal acquiescence, and this right necessarily forbids a physician or surgeon, however skillful or eminent . . . to violate without permission the bodily integrity of his patient . . . and [to operate] on him without his consent or knowledge.

Schloendorff v. The Society of New York Hospital (1914)

What Dr. Pratt had done to Mrs. Davis, another surgeon did nine years later to Mrs. Schloendorff. He removed a fibroid tumor even though she had insisted that ''there must be no operation.''[7] Mrs. Schloendorff had given permission for an examination under ether, but while ''unconscious a tumor was removed.'' Justice Cardozo first placed the legal issue in context: ''[i]n the case at hand, the wrong complained of is not merely negligence. It is trespass.'' Then he spoke with an economy of words about her right to self-determination, words that ever since have been incessantly quoted, particularly by those who ignore the fact situation in which they arose and instead seek to highlight his message of unfettered liberty: ''Every human being of adult years and sound mind has a right to determine what shall be done with his own body; and a surgeon who performs an operation without his patient's consent, commits an assault, for which he is liable in damages.''

A careful reading of *Pratt* and *Schloendorff*, however, does not bear out the sweeping contention that courts' pronouncements established patients' rights to ''thoroughgoing self-determination'' in interactions with their physicians. Consider the facts: Mrs. Schloendorff had repeatedly and vigorously opposed her operation and Mrs. Davis did not even know that a hysterectomy was contemplated. Both patients had been deliberately deceived about the nature of the intervention. Their bodily integrity had been invaded without any consent whatever, express or implied. These facts led Justices Cardozo and Brown to frame the disputes in trespass. And trespass, the forcible and uninvited entry into physical space—the disturbance of the "King's peace"— often evoked frightening memories in common law judges of invasions of land and home by marauders with their lances and spears. Trespass, in the cases before us, blended these ancient concerns with new ones that were equally disturbing: the invasion of abdomens and perinea by surgeons with their scalpels and knives. It was this fear—of something being done to persons, however medically appropriate, that they had not invited, indeed had vetoed—that judges wanted to allay with their uncompromising pronouncements, but no more than that.

Pratt and *Schloendorff* are memorable not for their pronouncements on self-determination—the egregious fact situations made such language unavoidable—but rather, for the necessity of having to remind physicians as late as this century's first and second decades of such elementary restraints on their professional authority in a democratic society. The physicians had said nothing about their intentions. Since the justices only wished to impose on doctors an absolute duty to advise patients of *what* was going to be done, they had an easy time saying what they did. That they also clothed their pronouncements in majestic and powerful language is equally true.

The cases neither invited nor required a sophisticated examination of the relationship between disclosure and consent, on the one hand, and self-determination, on the other. The asking of questions such as "how much do patients need to know in order to give meaningful consent" and "what must be communicated to and understood by patients to insure self-decision making," was still decades away. Until the mid-twentieth century, explicit legal protection of patients' right to choose was generally limited to instances in which physicians had performed surgery without permission. The disclosure requirement for purposes of valid consent and liberty was met as soon as patients had been informed of what the doctor intended to do.

In the few cases in which courts noted the inadequacy of disclosure, they viewed it not as an interference with patients' liberty and self-choice but as an inadvertent lapse from good care and custody, for which physicians ought not to be severely blamed. Courts tended to be as oblivious as physicians to the idea that inadequate disclosure made meaningful consent impossible and thus constituted an interference with patients' liberty.

Haskins v. Howard (1929)

Cases like *Haskins v. Howard*,[8] in which judges called for patient participation in decision making, were rare exceptions. Dr. Haskins had operated on Mrs. Maggie Howard despite doubts as to whether she was pregnant or suffering from an ovarian tumor. A miscarriage ensued. In upholding a jury verdict in favor of the patient, the appellate court noted not only the lack of good care and custody provided by the physician, who had acted "upon a too hasty, and therefore incomplete and improper, diagnosis," but also that "the consent of the patient or her husband to the operation was not obtained after a full disclosure of the doubt entertained by the defendant of the correctness of the diagnosis, and the hazard to be incurred." Yet, generally, evidence of inadequate disclosure was disregarded by courts. Indeed, plaintiffs and their attorneys unwittingly aided and abetted such judicial behavior, for they rarely thought of raising the allegation that a doctor had violated a patient's liberty. That allegation was not raised by Mrs. Howard, and even the court emphasized the importance of disclosure and consent only as an afterthought. The idea that patients had a role to play in medical decision making, beyond a mere right of refusal, rarely surfaced in judicial opinions during the reign of consent.

Hunt v. Bradshaw (1955)

Hunt v. Bradshaw[9] illustrates the disregard of, and the obliviousness to, both disclosure and consent. Sometime in 1950, John Hunt, hale and hearty, sustained an injury while working in his auto repair shop near Kingsport, Tennessee. A sledgehammer blow broke off a small, sharp-edged piece of steel, about 3/8" × 2/8" × 2/8", from the end of an automobile axle. It penetrated his body, entering the left front side of the neck just above his collar bone. A series of X-ray examinations revealed a small metal object, located 3/4" from the left lung and 4 1/2" from the heart. Dr. Bradshaw, a surgeon to whom Hunt had been referred, strongly recommended that it be removed. When Hunt inquired about the seriousness of the operation, Dr. Bradshaw supposedly responded that "it wasn't nothing to it (sic), it was very simple.'' Upon awakening from surgery, Hunt could no longer use his fingers. A claw hand on the left side remained his permanent legacy. The piece of metal was not recovered.

At the trial four years after the operation, two physicians, radiologist James Marr, and neurosurgeon Everett O. Jeffreys, testified on behalf of plaintiff. Dr. Marr limited his testimony to informing the jury that the piece of metal had hardly moved in the four years since the original injury. He noted that he had examined many X-rays displaying foreign objects lodged in the body and that they had been left there permanently without ill effects. ''The very best surgeons,'' Dr. Marr stated on the basis of considerable experience, ''frequently are unable to locate and remove small foreign bodies in the body of a patient.''

Dr. Jeffreys testified that injuries to nerves and arteries sustained during the operation were responsible for John Hunt's claw hand, that surgery generally was indicated and constituted good medical practice, that such small objects were often difficult to retrieve, and that he himself had had trouble finding them. In response to a hypothetical question, he declared that ''he would be inclined not to operate if the patient were free from symptoms—pain, temperature, etc.'' He added, that in his opinion, ''the patient should always be informed that he might have some disability from the arm [and about other salient points] as near as the doctor can tell him about what to expect, be it bad or be it good.''

No defense witnesses were called because, at the conclusion of plaintiff's presentation, the trial judge agreed with the defendant that plaintiff's case had failed for lack of expert testimony supporting an allegation of lack of due care either in performing the operation or in exercising good judgment in advising the patient about it. The case was dismissed.

Hunt appealed the verdict. Justice Higgins of the Tennessee Supreme Court affirmed the trial court's decision. He opined that plaintiff's expert witnesses had not cast sufficient doubt on Dr. Bradshaw's exercise of due care and of good judgment in his professional interactions with Hunt. He first noted that a physician ''is not civilly liable for [any untoward] consequences'' to his patient as long as he has ''professional learning, skill, and ability which others similarly situated ordinarily possess, [has exercised] reasonable care and diligence in the application of his knowledge and skill to the patient's case, [and has used] his best judgment in the treatment and care of his patient.''

With respect to the alleged lack of disclosure, the court simply stated:

> . . . It is understandable [that] the surgeon wanted to reassure the patient so that he would not go to the operating room unduly apprehensive. Failure to explain the risk involved, therefore, may be considered a mistake on the part of the surgeon, but under the facts cannot be deemed such want of ordinary care as to import liability.

In a brief concurring opinion Justice Bobbitt added:

> [T]he plaintiff alleges that when defendant recommended that the operation be performed, defendant *negligently* represented to him that the ''operation was a simple one which entailed and involved no danger to the plaintiff's health and body'' and that ''but for said representations . . . the plaintiff would not have submitted to said operation.'' But plaintiff did not allege that said representations were false to the knowledge of the defendant or other facts that might nullify his consent to the operation. In short, plaintiff's action is not for assault and battery, or trespass to the person, predicated upon allegations of an unauthorized operation.

Since such an action had not been brought, Justice Bobbitt concluded that it could not be determined whether ''plaintiff's evidence would [have been] sufficient for submission to the jury.''

Hunt v. Bradshaw is representative of the short shrift given to disclosure and consent as recently as the 1950's. Allegations of lack of adequate disclosure, if raised at all by plaintiff and his lawyer, were at best asserted peripherally, timidly, and almost inaudibly, for lawyers as well as their client-patients had grown up in, and had become accustomed to, a world in which doctors did not converse with patients. The emergence of novel and strange ideas such as informing patients about harmful consequences—information that might conceivably lead to a rejection of physicians' recommendations—could, to begin with, engender only anxious and contradictory doubts about patients' capacities to participate in decision making. Furthermore, the idea of challenging professionals' disclosure practices, of insisting on an informed consent, was equally unheard of. Its time had not yet come.

In addition, presenting evidence in support of the allegation of inadequate disclosure and consent encountered formidable obstacles. Plaintiffs and their lawyers appreciated the virtual impossibility of finding experts who would testify, in cases like *Hunt*, that a doctor's lack of candor had constituted bad professional practice. Without expert testimony that cast doubt on Dr. Bradshaw's exercise of "reasonable professional learning, reasonable care and reasonable judgment," he could not, as Justice Higgins correctly stated the law, be held "civilly liable." Indeed, such evidence could not have been introduced, however much Hunt's lawyer might have tried to locate expert witnesses, because a majority of physicians in Tennessee would have contended with unimpeachable honesty that not telling John Hunt about the risks of surgery and about alternatives was, if not good practice, at least the customary medical practice in Tennessee and elsewhere.

Put another way, even if some individual physicians in Tennessee had believed greater disclosure to be in the patient's best interests, on cross-examination they would also have been forced to admit that the majority of practicing physicians did not share the same view. Thus, under the existing rules of evidence and substantive law, Hunt had little chance of prevailing. Critics have often blamed a medical "conspiracy of silence" for the unavailability of experts to support plaintiff-patients' contentions in a court of law.[10] This is a mistaken belief. There is no conspiracy. Or, more accurately, if a conspiracy of silence exists, it takes place in the consulting room, right in front of the patient. It does not begin in a court of law before judge and jury. There the silence only speaks to the silence that years earlier pervaded the physician's office. What *Hunt* and many other cases of its day illustrate is that doctors did not talk to their patients and that neither physicians, nor judges, nor attorneys and their clients considered this surprising or odd.

Justice Bobbitt expressed some vague misgivings over the harm suffered by Hunt. He observed that medical treatment necessarily involved taking risks in order to bestow benefits; perhaps what had happened to Hunt could not have been avoided. But he wondered whether it was equally unavoidable for the law also to treat Hunt badly by not awarding him compensation for his injuries. His colleague, Justice Higgins, had already addressed and excused the medical dilemma over risks and benefits:

Of course, it seems hard to the patient in apparent good health that he should be advised to undergo an operation, and upon regaining consciousness find that he has lost the use of an arm for the remainder of his life. Infallibility in human beings is not attainable. The law recognizes, and we think properly so, that the surgeon's hand, with its skill and training, is, after all, a human hand, guided by a human brain in a procedure in which the margin between safety and danger sometimes measures little more than the thickness of a sheet of paper.

Justice Bobbitt, however, spoke to the legal dilemma. Hunt and his attorney had alleged that Dr. Bradshaw had "*negligently* represented to him that the 'operation was a simple one.' " Had Hunt and his attorney instead pleaded "assault and battery," Justice Bobbitt intimated, the case could perhaps have been submitted to a jury on the basis of facts that "might nullify [Hunt's] consent." Such comments brought no consolation to Hunt. Indeed, he could now only feel doubly damaged and wronged, first by an incompetent surgeon who perhaps had wrongly searched for a piece of steel and then by an incompetent lawyer who had pursued a wrong cause of action.

Justice Bobbitt's intimations were quite gratuitous, for Hunt's chances of succeeding in a battery action would have been exceedingly slim. The trial court probably would have ruled that a cause of action could not lie in battery because Hunt, after all, had been informed about the nature of the procedure and therefore had given at least his "implied consent." Or the appellate court would most likely have held, as another did when a physician had performed an esophagoscopy without the patient's "consent, express or implied," that such a "failure to obtain the patient's consent was unintentional . . . a mere oversight [and thus] did not constitute an 'assault and battery.' "[11] Recall that Justice Higgins also characterized Bradshaw's nondisclosures as a "mistake." Most likely, Justice Bobbitt's reference to an improper plea of the cause of action was merely an evasion to salve his own misgivings. Hunt would have failed under either cause of action.

Mistakes do happen. Fallibility is human. But much too little care has been taken in case law and scholarly commentary to distinguish not so much between avoidable and unavoidable accidents *per se*, but between potential accidents that have been jointly anticipated by physicians and their patients—a possible price to be paid for the promise of cure—and those that physicians either should have but did not anticipate, or if they did, had withheld from their patients.

A pervasive and significant blindspot in judicial thinking deserves emphasis. Courts' assertions that generally a failure to obtain consent is unintentional, an inadvertent "oversight," an occasional "mistake," and thus not "negligent," if taken at face value, are evidence of judicial ignorance about medical practices. An occasional lapse might be forgiven; but non-disclosure is not a mistake. It is, as I demonstrated in Chapter I, a systematic and intentional omission based upon deeply held professional beliefs that silence is in the patient's best interest.

Judges had to cling to the belief that physicians generally made disclosures that assured at least some measure of meaningful consent, for otherwise, they would have been forced to restructure radically physician-patient relations. This they were reluctant to do not only for reasons of unfamiliarity with the world of medicine but also out of an awareness, however dim, that it would prove enormously difficult to reconcile the medical with the jurisprudential world once they were forced to confront the problems of decision making between doctors and patients.

Perhaps judges also sensed that ordering sweeping changes in medical disclosure practices would affect the legal profession as well. After all, the relations of attorneys with clients do not differ significantly from those between physicians and patients. Judges' professional training, like that of their sibling-physicians, had socialized them to the virtues of the most minimal decision-making dialogue with clients. From their student days onward, they too had embraced the view that such professional conduct afforded clients' interest the best protection. Yet, as students of the common law, they had also been taught to respect citizens' rights to personal choice. They had tried to keep these two competing claims separate but, when citizen-patients' needs and rights clashed head-on, judges denied the pervasive disenfranchisement of patients in their decision-making interactions with doctors.

Thus, it is not surprising that by the mid 1950's, the judicial inquiry into the relationship between disclosure and consent, on the one hand, and self-determination, on the other, had not significantly advanced. Once physicians had been cautioned in *Pratt* and *Schloendorff* to tell patients what they planned to do, and to consider more carefully than they had in the past whether to proceed whenever patients objected to their proposed treatments, the courts rested for half a century. The rule of law in hospitals continued to be guided by principles of custody, not liberty.

The Birth and Development of Informed Consent

In the late 1950's judges began to ask a new, almost revolutionary, question: Are patients entitled not only *to know what* the doctor proposes to do but also *to decide whether* an intervention is acceptable in light of its risks and benefits and the available alternatives, including no treatment? The law of fraud and deceit, as Justice Bobbitt intimated in *Hunt*, had always protected patients from doctors' flagrant misrepresentations, and the law of battery had done the same for "unauthorized" interventions. Moreover, in theory, patients had always been entitled to ask whatever questions they pleased. What judges now groped toward was the proposition, eventually formalized in the doctrine of informed consent, that physicians should be placed under an *affirmative* duty to acquaint patients with the important risks and plausible alternatives to a proposed procedure.

Judges were hesitant to intrude on medical practices, and not only for reasons of unfamiliarity with the ways in which physicians worked. Their impulse to foster individual self-determination collided with an equally strong desire to maintain the authority of the profession, both for the sake of professionals and for the "best interests" of patients. The law had always respected the arcane expertise of physicians and rarely held them liable if they practiced "good medicine." These constraints made it impossible for the law of informed consent to advance patients' right to self-decision making in significant ways. Ultimately, concern over protecting patients' best interests by assuring them custody and care won out over protecting patients' self-determination and right to liberty.

This assessment of the current legal status of informed consent should not diminish an appreciation of the symbolic significance of the call for patient self-determination. However much courts might continue to try to evade, sidestep, and rationalize the complex questions informed consent poses, the new doctrine prevents them from banishing certain fundamental questions

completely from consciousness: Do patients have a voice in decisions affecting their medical lives? If so, what must a physician communicate so that patients' voices will not remain hollow
echoes?

Doctors and judges will have to learn to live at least with the
doctrine's symbolic significance. While it has always been the
fate of symbols to be honored more in words than in deeds, and
informed consent will prove to be no exception, symbols can nag
and prod and disturb and ultimately bring about some change.
The birth date of informed consent was 22 October 1957.
Twenty-six years is a brief moment in history, too short to bring
about significant changes in disclosure and consent, particularly
since human beings have always had a difficult time learning to
communicate with one another. It will take time for physicians
and patients to make the slow ascent, if they will make it at all,
from their feudal past.

Salgo v. Leland Stanford Jr. University Board of Trustees (1957)

The doctrine of informed consent surfaced, seemingly out of nowhere, in *Salgo v. Leland Stanford Jr. University Board of Trustees.*[12]
The way Justice Bray of the California Court of Appeals introduced it in a brief paragraph at the end of his opinion made me
recall Greek plays, the final appearance of the *deus ex machina,*
who miraculously resolved all the human predicaments that the
playwright had tried to address.

Where had the doctrine come from? I could unearth no ante-
cedent cases. In an earlier article [13] I speculated somewhat fanci-
fully that Justice Bray, after reflecting before going to sleep on
the opinion he would write the next morning, had perhaps
dreamed of the phrase "informed consent." For there is a
dreamlike quality to the informed consent part of the opinion,
both in the way it was introduced and in its language. But the answer is less fanciful and at the same time more intriguing. The
entire informed consent paragraph in *Salgo* was adopted verba-
tim, and without attribution, from the *amicus curiae* brief submitted by the American College of Surgeons to the California Court
of Appeals.[14] It is an ironic twist of history that informed consent,
so bitterly opposed by most physicians, was dreamed up by lawyers in the employ of doctors.

The events that precipitated the legal controversy in *Salgo* had occurred a number of years earlier. Martin Salgo, 55-years-old, had been suffering for some years from cramping pains in his leg and intermittent limping. His doctor suspected a block in his abdominal aorta and recommended the performance of an aortography in order to locate the block. The procedure required the injection of a dye, sodium urokon. In 1954, aortography had not "been used enough in the bay area to constitute routine procedure."[15] When Salgo awoke the morning after the procedure, he could not move his legs. He claimed that the permanent paralysis of his lower extremities was due to the negligent performance of the translumbar aortography by the doctors on the staff of the Stanford University Hospital. He later appended a claim that the physicians negligently had failed to warn him of the risks of paralysis inherent in the procedure. Justice Bray reversed the trial court's judgment for the defendants on a number of grounds, including errors by the trial court in giving instructions to the jury concerning physicians' duty to warn of the risk of paralysis.

Justice Bray's opening pronouncements on informed consent were quite emphatic (although the words were those submitted by the American College of Surgeons, I shall refer to them as Justice Bray's since he adopted them and gave them legal force): "A physician violates his duty to his patient and subjects himself to liability if he withholds any facts which are necessary to form the basis of an intelligent consent by the patient to the proposed treatment." But he immediately had second thoughts, revolving around two questions: How much should doctors disclose to avoid the danger of unfairly inducing a patient's consent, and how much should doctors withhold to avoid the danger of alarming an already apprehensive patient even more?

Justice Bray found answers to his questions in a charmed new phrase, "informed consent," which appeared at the end of a most ambiguous sentence: "[I]n discussing the element of risk a certain amount of discretion must be employed consistent with the full disclosure of facts necessary to an informed consent." This was a startling piece of work. Going in two opposite directions—discretion and full disclosure—his answer went nowhere. Yet, even if *Salgo* did not clarify the law, at least it stimulated a great debate.

Before I discovered the origins of Justice Bray's informed consent language I thought that, in simply announcing an absolute duty to disclose all the "facts which are necessary to form the basis of an intelligent consent," he had intended to give greater legal protection to a patient's right of self-determination. I speculated that the court, sensing the immense difficulty that judges would encounter if they had to set forth in absolute and general terms what these facts might be, quickly bowed to the "discretion" and "experience" of the medical profession. I also noted that in delegating unspecified discretion to the medical profession to make judgments about patients' self-determination, the court did not appreciate the futility of its endeavors, for it gave an undefined task to a group that has had neither the experience with nor the commitment to patient self-determination.

While such conflicting considerations may still have moved Justice Bray to adopt the language of the *amicus* brief, the discovery of the brief submitted by the American College of Surgeons suggests another, and better, speculation of what transpired at the time of informed consent's birth. When *Salgo* was being appealed, representatives of the American College of Surgeons must have met with their attorneys to discuss the scope of the *amicus* brief that they intended to submit to Justice Bray. It seems likely that then the total silence of the physicians in the face of a new, powerful, and hazardous technology cast a dark, uncomfortable shadow over their deliberations.

Recall that the *Pratt* and *Schloendorff* opinions originated out of judicial concern that the increasing employment of anesthesia could lead to chloroformed consent, to giving physicians license to proceed without even telling patients what they intended to do to them. It was the *total* etherized silence that had disturbed Justices Brown and Cardozo then. This same silence may have made the surgeons and their attorneys uncomfortable when they began talking with one another about how to justify the silent treatment of Mr. Salgo. The silence would also disturb Justice Bray, and three years later Justice Schroeder in *Natanson v. Kline*,[16] the first opinion to construe informed consent in some depth.

It is one thing to interact silently with patients at the bedside; it is another to confess to the silence away from the bedside. The silence then becomes deafeningly loud. Most likely, the surgeons and their attorneys talked haltingly and wearily with one another about the need to remain silent so that patients would not become more apprehensive than they already were. But the doctors may have had a difficult time defining when and why they kept silent. Silence in physician-patient relations had been undiscriminatingly accepted for too long to allow for meaningful distinctions. Perhaps the lawyers, in observing their clients' discomfort, began to realize that they, though more used to talking to their clients than physicians to their patients, also left much unsaid and exercised much greater silent control over their clients' legal fate than they had appreciated. For long moments the lawyers and physicians must have been quite uncomfortable with one another.

Thus it is not surprising that the informed consent part of the *Salgo* opinion has all the eyemarks of a dream, though not one originally dreamed by Justice Bray, as I once thought, but one elaborated by the surgeons and lawyers in the twilight of their deliberations. At first glance, the *amicus* brief made the same kind of sense as a dream from which one has just awakened. In dreams, one can arrange a peace treaty between Hannibal and Garibaldi without an awareness of its historical impossibility, and even remain convinced of having accomplished that feat for a while after awakening, until critical judgment returns. Similarly, only self-conscious reflection can make it clear that such contradictory intentions as "full disclosure of facts" and "[professional] discretion" are reconcilable only in the kingdom of dreams. Upon awakening, modifications become necessary, and the appearance of such qualifying words as "a certain amount of discretion" reveals the ego at work, reconciling the contradictions, attempting to give both their just due by the least painful compromise.

Justice Bray was troubled by the facts of the case, as Justice Schroeder would be later in *Natanson*. The novel and awe-inspiring medical procedures—aortography in *Salgo* and cobalt radiation in *Natanson*—had injured rather than healed. Both justices must have felt that, since the employment of the new technologies not only promised great benefits but also could expose patients to formidable and uncontrollable risks, they should not be administered to patients without prior conversation. Here the justices might have been influenced by a line of cases, dating back at least to 1767, in which courts had warned physicians that, whenever they used new and as yet untried interventions, they did so "at their peril."[17] They had instructed doctors, whenever they employed such "*experimental*" procedures, to do so "with the knowledge and consent of the patient or those responsible for him."[18]

Yet, Justice Bray must have recognized the inadequacy of existing malpractice law to resolve the problems created by the advances in modern technology. Something new had happened to the practice of medicine. The potential harm of these novel interventions seemed to demand a reappraisal of the traditional prerogatives of professionals and of the rights and needs of patients. Thus the *amicus* brief, submitted on behalf of a most distinguished group of surgeons, might well have delighted Justice Bray. At least it acknowledged a patient's right to know. Indeed, it was one of the few documents he had received, and none as authoritative, that had addressed the duty to disclose. He might have sensed that an effort to improve on its language would lead to trouble, to an awareness of the contradictions inherent in the brief before him. Thus it seemed better not to tamper with it.

I have employed the dream analogy deliberately in order to suggest that any deceptions that occurred during the birth of informed consent were not designed to deceive others—for example, the appellate judge—but rather, constituted a deception of self. The participants deceived themselves into believing that disclosure and discretion could readily be reconciled, that they did not have to take great care to prevent discretion from swallowing disclosure—a danger particularly great in professional settings. Put another way, in juxtaposing wishes for disclosure and discretion as if they were non-rivalrous siblings, the surgeons and their attorneys unselfconsciously and unreflectively avoided the necessity of facing up to the painful reality of conflict in their interactions with patients and of learning how to accommodate to this reality.

Physicians and lawyers did not appreciate that an inquiry into the scope of informed consent would lead to a confrontation with the conflict-ridden nature of man, to a realization that conflicts within and between human beings are never totally resolvable; that the interests of physicians and patients rarely coincide. The idea that physicians' and patients' interests are one and the same allows a doctor to speak for the patient. That idea has been the bedrock of physician-patient relations since the beginning of time. Recall the words of Ludmilla Afanasyevna that "without a physician's right to make decisions for the patient, there'd be no such thing as medicine."[19] There will always be medicine. The question that begs for an answer is: Can a new medicine be built on a foundation dedicated to the idea that patients also have a right to make decisions?

The final verdict on *Salgo* is this: The opinion left the law of disclosure and consent utterly confused. It opened the door, however, for judges to apply evolving jurisprudential pronouncements on privacy and self-determination from other areas of law to physician-patient controversies. It raised the issue of how much freedom of choice to grant patients. It gave rise to the question, "should patients be charged with responsibility for their own mistakes?" Thus *Salgo* initiated a process that eventually could force medicine to abandon its feudal practices. That little has happened since *Salgo* is not a sign of failure; 26 years is too short a time to bring about significant changes in a 2000-year-old tradition of silence. For Justice Bray to have initiated such a process is an achievement in its own right.

Natanson v. Kline (1960)

The next development in the doctrine of informed consent occurred in 1960, when the Kansas Supreme Court decided *Natanson v. Kline*.[20] Justice Schroeder's opinion established the law on disclosure and consent for the next 12 years in almost all jurisdictions that considered the matter. Subsequent to a mastectomy, Mrs. Irma Natanson suffered injuries from cobalt therapy employed to reduce the risks that her breast cancer would recur or spread. She sued Dr. John R. Kline, her radiologist, claiming both that he had been negligent in the administration of treatment and that he had failed to advise her of the nature of the proposed treatment and its hazards. The injuries were severe. One of the attorneys described them to me, years after the trial, in vivid language:

> I have been in many trials, but this one was one of the most dramatic of my experience. The plaintiff's attorneys proposed as part of the plaintiff's evidence that the burned area be exhibited to the jury. The request was granted by the trial judge and so the courtroom was closed to the public and all spectators (if any) were excluded. The curtains were drawn and Mrs. Natanson who was an attractive woman bared herself to the waist and all could see the injury. As I recall it, the mastectomy site was on the left side. Beneath

it, the ribs had been destroyed by the radiation and the best that Dr. Brown had been able to accomplish, was to have a layer of skin over the opening. I recall seeing the beat of the heart reflected in movements of this skin flap. The burned area as I remember it over the years, was shaped somewhat like a football, although smaller. The longest axis was vertical and the total area was probably about 8 inches x 4 inches.[21]

The trial court declined plaintiff's request to instruct the jury on the duty of physicians to warn patients of treatment hazards, but the Kansas Supreme Court reversed the decision, specifying that physicians had "the obligation . . . to disclose and explain to the patient in language as simple as necessary the nature of the ailment, the probability of success or of alternatives, and perhaps the risks of unfortunate results and unforeseen conditions within the body."[22]

Justice Schroeder, writing for the court, based the new requirement on a fundamental jurisprudential principle:

Anglo-American law starts with the premise of thorough-going self-determination. It follows that each man is considered to be master of his own body, and he may, if he be of sound mind, expressly prohibit the performance of life-saving surgery, or other medical treatment. A doctor might well believe that an operation or form of treatment is desirable or necessary but the law does not permit him to substitute his own judgment for that of the patient by any form of artifice or deception.

Before setting forth its new rule, and the premise on which it was based, the court noted that it had not found a Kansas case that addressed the extent of physicians' duties "to explain the nature and probable consequences of that treatment [and to] disclose the existence and nature of the risks inherent in the treatment." With the exception of *Salgo* which the court quoted in detail, adopting its "proper rule," none of the cases from foreign jurisdictions were "directly on point." In the annals of law, *Natanson* was a case of first impression.

In enumerating specific disclosure obligations, and in finding the roots of these obligations in Anglo-American law's "premise of thorough-going self-determination," *Natanson* made more explicit what had been foreshadowed in *Salgo*. Although Justice Schroeder's pronouncements on disclosure were a radical departure from what judges had said in the past, implementation of both the disclosure obligation and the noble underlying premise was riddled with ambiguities and ultimately quite limited. After some of the ambiguities were pointed out to him by the defense lawyers, Justice Schroeder issued another opinion, the second in an attempt "to clarify" the first opinion. He did not succeed, in part because he made incorrect assumptions about the nature of medical practices concerning disclosure and consent. In addition, when faced with problems of implementing the principle of "thorough-going self-determination," he compromised it in favor of medical paternalism.

Justice Schroeder's opening moves signaled that *Natanson* would not significantly advance the decision-making rights of patients. After reciting the facts of the case, he directed his attention to the defendant's contention that since Mrs. Natanson had "consented" to cobalt radiation, "this is not an action for assault and battery, where a patient has given *no* consent to the treatment." The court did not address this argument directly and instead introduced puzzling distinctions between unauthorized treatments and battery:

> What appears to distinguish the case of the unauthorized surgery or treatment from traditional assault and battery cases is the fact that in almost all the cases the physician is acting in relatively good faith for the benefit of the patient. . . . The traditional assault and battery involves a defendant who is acting for the most part out of malice or in a manner generally considered as "antisocial." One who commits an assault and battery is not seeking to confer any benefit upon the one assaulted.
>
> The fundamental distinction between assault and battery on the one hand, and negligence such as would constitute malpractice, on the other, is that the former is intentional and the latter unintentional.

Justice Schroeder tried his best to avoid calling this a case of battery. He employed the label "unauthorized treatment" instead, because Mrs. Natanson had known about and submitted to the treatment. At the same time, there was no controversy—Dr. Kline pleaded lack of memory—over plaintiff's contention that the doctor had said nothing at all about the hazard of cobalt radiation, which was a new treatment modality in Wichita, Kansas, in 1955. Even though Justice Schroeder concluded that "[u]pon the record here presented Dr. Kline made no disclosures to [Mrs. Natanson] whatever,'' he was reluctant to employ the language of *Pratt* and *Schloendorff* for such an ''unauthorized'' treatment. His reluctance to invoke the language of trespass was due to the fact that, unlike Mrs. Davis or Mrs. Schloendorff, Mrs. Natanson had agreed to the proposed treatment. He did not confront the issue that her consent was meaningless since a crucial fact—the dangers of cobalt radiation—had been kept from her. Instead he made spurious distinctions between different kinds of assault and battery, which allowed him to come to the conclusion that what Dr. Kline had done was not a battery but negligence. Of course, there were other reasons as well: for example, the court would have been most uncomfortable calling Dr. Kline a ''trespasser'' or ''batterer.''

Justice Schroeder's preference for negligence over battery as a cause of action reflected a misreading of the law of battery and a misunderstanding of medical practices. With respect to the law of battery, law professors Fowler V. Harper and Fleming James, Jr., long ago emphasized that to allege battery, ''the intention need not be malicious, nor need it be an intention to inflict actual damage. It is sufficient if the actor intends to inflict either a harmful or offensive contact without the other's consent or to put the other in apprehension thereof.''[23] These authorities made it quite clear that while ''intent'' is required for a defendant's conduct to constitute a battery, ''it is only necessary to establish (a) that the actor engage in volitional activity and (b) that he intend to violate the legally protected interest of another in his person.''

Even if it were granted, as it should be, that Dr. Kline did not and that physicians generally do not act out of ''malice'' but ''in relatively good faith for the benefit of the patient,'' such good faith and beneficence are immaterial if the medical intervention was carried out without consent, if ''it violates a legally protected interest of another in his person.'' In *Natanson* Justice Schroeder substituted the *colloquial* meaning of ''malice'' for its *legal* meaning. Clearly by deliberately withholding information from Mrs. Natanson, Dr. Kline and his Kansas colleagues, as admitted in the *amicus* brief of the Kansas Medical Society, did what they had always done, with full knowledge, in the exercise of sound professional judgment and irrespective of any contrary requirement of law. Thus, Dr. Kline's professional conduct, indeed, the conduct of the entire medical profession, was ''anti-social'' in its legal meaning.

The ambivalence of Justice Schroeder toward patient self-determination manifested itself strikingly in the competition between battery and negligence. In subsequent informed consent cases across the country the same conflict was almost always resolved in favor of negligence law—a cause of action more favorable to physicians—disguising a basic policy choice between patients' self-determination and doctor's paternalism as a choice between battery and negligence.

Judges have rejected battery for a number of reasons. Battery is an uncompromising remedy, allowing few defenses. Judges have feared that its adoption would give too much advantage to the plaintiff-patient. As one authority widely quoted in case law observed:

> A physician sued in a battery case has relatively little "elbow room" in which to establish a defense. A physician sued for medical negligence in failing to disclose hazards has many possibilities on which to base a defense under the circumstances that existed. Herein lies one of the significant practical reasons why the distinctions [between battery and negligence] should be kept intact.[24]

In deference to the mysteries of medicine, judges have based the legal standard of physicians' behavior on actual medical practices rather than on judicial theory, and battery law traditionally has not relied on a professional standard of care. Expansion of the requisites for valid consent within the ambit of battery would have reduced the need for medical testimony in deciding consent controversies, and thus would have limited the impact on the legal process of physicians' beliefs about what patients are entitled to know.

The choice of negligence theory allowed judges to defer gracefully to medical judgment, permitting physicians to continue to exercise the wisdom of their profession and making them liable only for failure to disclose what a typical, and hence, reasonable doctor would have revealed under the circumstances. Negligence law places additional burdens on patients by requiring proof that they would have refused the proposed treatment if they had been fully informed. Furthermore, negligence law generally does not redress dignitary injuries in the absence of physical injury. It leaves little room for the idea that lack of disclosure should be a legally cognizable injury in and of itself. Instead, the law of informed consent should compensate all interferences with self-determination regardless of their impact on the patients' decision or physical health.

Justice Schroeder's ultimate retreat to traditional negligence law was so complete that the paragraph on self-determination stands all alone, surrounded by words that repudiate its meaning. The paragraph on self-determination has an interesting history all its own. Justice Schroeder had been unable to find any legal precedent, except in *Salgo*, for a duty to disclose. He eventually "found" it in a law journal article, authored by Hubert Winston Smith,[25] a physician-lawyer. He adopted Smith's language without attribution.

The court was caught on the horns of a dilemma. Justice Schroeder intuitively appreciated that disclosure and consent, if they made any sense, had to be based on a right of patients to participate in decision making, that is, on self-determination. Therefore, he had to establish some standards for disclosure from the patient's vantage point. Once having taken this small step, however, he became concerned about whether the modest standards of disclosure that he had established had been too great a leap. Fearing that logic had gotten the better of "common sense," which dictated leaving decision making to doctors, he invoked the professional standard of care and the therapeutic privilege to withhold information as counterweights:

> The duty of the physician to disclose, however, is limited to those disclosures which a reasonable medical practitioner would make under the same or similar circumstances. How the physician may best discharge his obligation to the patient in this difficult situation involves primarily a question of medical judgment.
>
> *   *   *
>
> There is probably a privilege, on therapeutic grounds, to withhold the specific diagnosis where the disclosure of cancer or some other dread disease would seriously jeopardize the recovery of an unstable, temperamental or severely depressed patient.[26]

Since physicians were not committed to sharing the burdens of decision with patients, recourse to the professional standard of disclosure and invocation of a vaguely worded therapeutic privilege not to disclose could only stifle the court's call for self-determination. Thus Justice Schroeder, in not permitting the eloquent words on "thorough-going self-determination" to inform the rest of his opinion, created new tensions that have plagued the informed consent doctrine ever since.

Grafting sturdy branches of negligence law on a slender root of self-determination could not propogate a vigorous hybrid doctrine that would thrive in a climate traditionally inhospitable to patients' participation in decision making. Justice Schroeder had good intentions, but good intentions, particularly if one is ambivalent toward them, have a devil of a time in unwelcome settings.

Canterbury v. Spence (1972)

Judge Robinson, of the D.C. Court of Appeals, who authored the next and last landmark informed consent decision, also had good intentions. Although the opinion of *Canterbury v. Spence*[27] is an improvement over that of *Natanson*, ultimately he too failed, as Justice Schroeder had before him, to advance patients' rights to self-determination significantly.

The grounds for this failure are not to be found in policy considerations alone—in a felt necessity, for example, for the law of torts to balance such competing needs as safeguarding patients' rights to self-determination with physicians' and their insurers' rights to economic well-being. The causes of failure are deeply buried in doubts about patients' capacities to make reasonable decisions and in fears that meddling with unquestioned faith will undermine cure. Judges have had some awareness of these competing considerations. It has blunted their commitment to patients' rights and made them wary of going beyond a symbolic gesture, of providing much needed guidance on how to translate rhetoric into practice. Whatever meager direction they had given became readily enmeshed in contradiction and confusion.

One can contend that seminal opinions like *Natanson* and *Canterbury* should not be expected to articulate in detail something as complex as a doctrine of informed consent; or that courts, in any case, can only make general pronouncements to prod professionals gradually to change their practices. Whatever the merits of such contentions, they do not invalidate the lesson to be learned from a study of *Canterbury*: The strong commitment to self-determination at the beginning of the opinion gets weaker as the opinion moves from jurisprudential theory to the realities of hospital and courtroom life. By the end, the opinion has only obscured the issue it intended to address: the nature of the relationship between the court's doctrine of informed consent, as ultimately construed, and its root premise of self-determination.

In 1959, 19-year-old Mr. Canterbury underwent a laminectomy for severe back pain. After the operation, he apparently recuperated uneventfully for a day. Needing to urinate and with no one around to assist him, he tried to fend for himself. He fell out of bed and suffered "an almost immediate setback." Within a few hours he could not move his legs and soon thereafter, he became paralyzed from the waist down. This paralysis still persisted in 1972, when Judge Robinson rendered his opinion. Plaintiff sued Dr. Spence for negligent performance of a laminectomy and later appended to this basic claim the allegation of negligent failure to warn of the risks of paralysis.*

Clearly Judge Robinson's heart went out to young Canterbury and his physical plight: "[t]he record we review tells a depressing tale. A youth troubled only by back pain . . . [now] hobble[s] about on crutches, a victim of paralysis of the bowels and urinary incontinence." Judge Robinson's mind was also disturbed by the lack of informed consent: "A youth troubled only by back pain submitted to an operation without being informed of a risk of paralysis incidental thereto. . . . In a very real sense this lawsuit is an *understandable search for reasons*."

The court started again from the venerable idea of self-determination: "The root premise is the concept, fundamental in American jurisprudence, that '[e]very human being of adult years and sound mind has a right to determine what shall be done with his own body.' " These were the words of Justice Cardozo in *Schloendorff*, and to them Judge Robinson added his own: "[t]rue consent to what happens to one's self is the informed exercise of a choice, and that entails an opportunity to evaluate knowledgeably the options available and the risks attendant upon each."

Recall, that Cardozo's root premise was articulated in a case

*Since Canterbury's paralysis may have been the result of an accident subsequent to surgery, the fact situation of *Canterbury v. Spence* makes it an ill-suited case for the courts to have used in spelling out the disclosure obligations of physicians. Facts notwithstanding, *Canterbury* has become a landmark decision in the legal history of informed consent.

in which a patient allegedly had been operated on without her knowledge or her consent. It was easier in 1917, as it is still today, to treat such uninvited interventions, even if perpetrated by physicians, as battery, to condemn them as an unpardonable disrespect of citizen-patients' right to self-determination. But, when physicians have made some disclosure and patients have given some consent, questions arise: How much disclosure constitutes "disclosure"? What quality of consent constitutes "consent"? Few courts have been willing to explore these questions and to specify when disclosure becomes so inadequate that consent is spurious in law. The bold opinion of one court that "[if] the lack of sufficient information vitiates a consent the cause of action is the same as if no consent had ever been given,"[28] was quickly overruled.[29]

Although the *Canterbury* court rejected battery and grounded the disclosure requirement in negligence law, as the *Natanson* court had done 12 years earlier, it observed that "due care normally demands that the physician warn the patient of *any* risks to his well-being which contemplated therapy may involve."[30] Judge Robinson supported his choice by noting that the duty to warn is "surely a facet of due care." Since "due care" is firmly embedded in negligence law, ergo negligence law clearly applied.

Judge Robinson recognized the dilemma that his posited duty created in negligence law. Though courts in many jurisdictions had announced such a duty to disclose, they left it in a legal limbo by requiring plaintiffs to establish the prevailing duty to disclose through expert testimony, based on professional standards. The obligations to disclose promulgated by the courts thus mattered little at trial, since physicians were substantially allowed to make their own law with respect to disclosure. Judge Robinson seemed to address this problem squarely by eliminating the professional standard of practice with respect to disclosure:

> There are, in our view, formidable obstacles to acceptance of the notion that the physician's obligation to disclose is either germinated or limited by medical practice. To begin with, the reality of any discernible custom reflecting a professional consensus on communication of option and risk information to patients is open to serious doubt. We sense the danger that what in fact is no custom at all may be taken as an affirmative custom to maintain silence. . . .

> Respect for the patient's right of self-determination on particular
> therapy demands a standard set by law for physicians rather than
> one which physicians may or may not impose upon themselves.

For this apparently bold move, *Canterbury* has been widely celebrated, as well as followed in many jurisdictions.

The new rule of law laid down in *Canterbury*, however, is far
from clear. Judge Robinson, returning to basic principles of expert testimony, simply said that there is "no basis for operation
of the special medical standard where the physician's activity
does not bring his medical knowledge and skills peculiarly into
play," and that ordinarily disclosure is not such a situation. But
he left room for such situations by adding: "When medical judgment enters the picture and for that reason the special standard
controls, prevailing medical practice must be given its *just due*."
He did not spell out the meaning of "*just due*."

Both standards tend to confuse the need for *medical knowledge*
to elucidate the risks of and alternatives to a proposed procedure
in the light of professional experience with the need for *medical
judgment* to establish the limits of appropriate disclosure to patients. The difference is crucial to the clarification of the law of
informed consent. In *Natanson* and many subsequent cases,
judges lumped the two together uncritically, relying solely on
current medical practice to resolve the question of reasonableness
of disclosure. In *Canterbury*, the distinction was formally recognized. The plaintiff was required to present expert evidence of
the applicable medical knowledge, while the defendant had to
raise the issue of medical judgment to limit disclosure in defense.
But even *Canterbury* did not undertake a detailed judicial analysis
of the nature of medical judgment required, precisely because
judges were hesitant to make rules in an area that doctors
strongly believed was solely the province of medicine.

In *Canterbury*, Dr. Spence claimed that "communication of
that risk (paralysis) to the patient is not good medical practice because it might deter patients from undergoing needed surgery
and might produce adverse psychological reactions which could
preclude the success of the operation." Such claims will almost
invariably be raised by physicians since they are derived from
deeply held tenets of medical practice. Judge Robinson's enig-
matic phrase of "just due" certainly suggests that the medical
professional standard would be applicable in such a case, raising

profound questions about the extent to which the novel legal standard has been swallowed up by the traditional and venerable medical standard.

In fact, medical judgment was given its "just due" twice. It could also be invoked under the "therapeutic privilege" not to disclose, which Judge Robinson retained as a defense to disclosure:

> It is recognized that patients occasionally become so ill or emotionally distraught on disclosure as to foreclose a rational decision, or complicate or hinder the treatment, or perhaps even pose psychological damage to the patient. . . . The critical inquiry is whether the physician responded to a sound medical judgment that communication of the risk information would present a threat to the patient's well-being.

The therapeutic privilege not to disclose is merely a procedurally different way of invoking the professional standard of care. Once the physician has produced evidence that the failure to disclose represented a reasonable exercise of medical judgment, it is unclear whether the plaintiff-patient must introduce expert testimony to the contrary. If so, then there is virtually no difference between the *Natanson* and *Canterbury* lines of cases, since the plaintiff will almost always be obliged to produce expert testimony that non-disclosure was unreasonable.

In elaborating on the new legal standard for disclosure, the *Canterbury* court was compelled to go further than previous courts had in tracing the ramifications of that standard. Since the court wished to depart from medical custom as the standard, it had to give some indication as to the information it expected physicians to disclose. The court said that "the test for determining whether a particular peril must be divulged is its materiality to the patient's decision: all risks potentially affecting the decision must be unmasked." It added that physicians must similarly disclose alternatives to the proposed treatment and the "results likely if the patient remains untreated."

But then the court chose to adopt an "objective" test for disclosure of risks and alternatives—"what a [reasonable] *prudent* person in the patient's position would have decided if suitably informed"—and rejected a "subjective" test of materiality— "what an *individual* patient would have considered a significant risk." In opting for an "objective" standard, self-determination was given unnecessarily short shrift. The whole point of the inquiry was to safeguard the right of *individual* choice, even where it may appear idiosyncratic. Although law generally does not protect a person's right to be unreasonable and requires reasonably prudent conduct where injury to another may occur, it remains ambiguous about the extent to which prudence can be legally enforced where the potential injury is largely confined to the individual decision maker. For example, courts have split on the question of whether society may require the wearing of motorcycle helmets[31] and whether an adult patient may be compelled to undergo unwanted blood transfusions.[32]

The "objective" standard for disclosure contradicts the right of each individual to decide what will be done with his or her body. The belief that there is one "reasonable" or "prudent" response to every situation inviting medical intervention is nonsense, from the point of view of both the physician and the patient. The most cursory examination of medical practices demonstrates that what is reasonable to the internist may appear unreasonable to the surgeon or even to other internists and, more significantly, that the value preferences of physicians may not coincide with those of their patients. For example, doctors generally place a higher value on physical longevity than their patients do. But physical longevity is not the only touchstone of prudence. Why should not informed consent law countenance a wide range of potentially reasonable responses by patients to their medical condition based on other value preferences?

Since different doctors often approach similar cases in vastly dissimilar ways, why should not equally varying responses by patients be considered "reasonable"? After all, the aim of the doctrine is not to encourage uniformity in medical treatment, but to preserve individual choice. Yet most courts, while doing rhetorical honors to self-determination, have adopted this self-contradictory position. One exception is the Oklahoma Supreme Court. In *Scott v. Bradford*, Justice Doolin observed:

> [T]he *Canterbury* . . . "reasonable man" approach has been criticized . . . as backtracking on its own theory of self-determination. The *Canterbury* view certainly severely limits the protection granted an injured patient. To the extent the plaintiff, given an adequate disclosure, would have declined the proposed treatment, and a reasonable person in similar circumstances would have consented, a

patient's right of self-determination is *irrevocably lost*. This basic right to know and decide is the reason for the full-disclosure rule. Accordingly, we decline to jeopardize this right by the imposition of the "reasonable man" standard.[33]

Justice Doolin recognized that if the grand rhetoric of self-determination is to have meaning, framing the question in terms of the decision of a reasonable person grossly and unnecessarily substitutes judicial paternalism at a critically wrong point.

Although Justice Robinson appreciated that a "subjective" test of materiality was more in keeping with the right of self-determination than the "reasonable man" approach, he rejected it for fear that such a test would unfairly burden physicians by requiring them to guess the needs of particular patients. Thus he ruled that a physician should be compelled to divulge only that information required by "the average reasonable patient":

> Of necessity, the content of the disclosure rests in the first instance with the physician. Ordinarily it is only he who is in position to identify particular dangers; always he must make a judgment, in terms of materiality, as to whether and to what extent revelation to the patient is called for. He cannot know with complete exactitude what the patient would consider important to his decision, but on the basis of his medical training and experience he can sense how the average, reasonable patient expectably would react. Indeed, with knowledge of, or ability to learn, his patient's background and current condition, he is in a position superior to that of most others—attorneys, for example—who are called upon to make judgments on pain of liability in damages for unreasonable miscalculation.[34]

Despite the court's urging to be attentive to the needs of patients in the disclosure process, it all too readily allayed any worries about making "an undue demand upon medical practitioners" on matters of disclosure by endowing them with the capacity to divine what their patients wanted to hear. The court's emphasis on "sensing" the needs of particular patients, for example, invites the withholding of information as an exercise of therapeutic discretion. But physicians cannot know with *any* exactitude what patients will consider important, and little in their medical training and experience prepares them, if it ever could, to sense how patients will react to disclosures. Here again, a court rendered an opinion based on a complete misconception of the nature of medical practice. The court quickly disregarded the implication of what it had correctly asserted earlier: "[T]he reality of any discernible custom reflecting a professional consensus on communication of option and risk information to patients is open to serious doubt." If there is no "custom," how can there be "training and experience"?

The art of conversing with patients has to be painstakingly learned. When the court compared the disclosure and consent processes in law with those in medicine, it may have appreciated this fact for a moment. But again, by placing physicians in "a position superior to that of . . . attorneys," the court dismissed the complex communication problems that disclosure and consent raise for all professions. Lawyers have the same "knowledge of, or ability to learn [their clients'] background and current condition," as doctors have. What Judge Robinson, trained as a lawyer, knew to be difficult for attorneys, he should have known to be equally difficult for physicians.

Ascertaining patients' informational needs is difficult. Answers do not lie in guessing or "sensing" patients' particular concerns or in obliterating the "subjective" person in an "objective" mass of persons. The "objective" test of materiality only tempts doctors to introduce their own unwarranted subjectivity into the disclosure process. It would have been far better if the court had not committed itself prematurely to the labels "objective" and "subjective." Instead it should have considered more the patients' plight and required physicians to learn new skills: how to inquire openly about their patients' *individual* informational needs and patients' concerns, doubts, and misconceptions about treatment—its risks, benefits, and alternatives. Safeguarding self-determination requires assessing whether patients' informational needs have been satisfied by asking them whether they understand what has been explained to them. Physicians should not try to "second-guess" patients or "sense" how they will react. Instead, they need to explore what questions require further explanation. Taking such unaccustomed obligations seriously is not easy.

Indeed, the court's emphasis on specific disclosures, particularly of material risks, reinforces the traditional passive mode of patients' interactions with their doctors. Risk information, like everything else patients need to know, can become meaningful to patients only if they are viewed as active participants in decision making. In its discussion on materiality, for example, the court emphasized the responsibility of the physician to "make a *judgment* in terms of materiality." In other words, it focused on what should be told *to*, rather than discussed *with*, patients. Autonomous decision making requires two-way conversation.

The *Canterbury* court, in agreement with the *Natanson* court, accepted the traditional requirement that the undisclosed risk must materialize in order to establish liability. The court added sadly, "otherwise the omission, however unpardonable, is legally without consequence." It then went on to explain, "[o]ccurrence of the risk must be harmful to the patient, for negligence unrelated to injury is nonactionable."

This explanation, however pertinent to negligence law, demonstrates strikingly how far the court had strayed from its root premise. Interferences with self-determination occur in all situations in which a person's dignitary interests have been violated. They are not limited to those in which physical harm has occurred. Lack of informed consent is itself a violation. It is the harm. The additional presence of physical harm only adds injury to insult.

The *Canterbury* court also required proof that the disclosure of the risk to the patient would have resulted in "altered conduct," that is, in a decision against the proposed treatment. This requirement should be eliminated because it conflicts with respect for the dignity of the individual and the right to self-determination. As citizens, patients are wronged when physicians begin treatment without fulfilling their disclosure obligation. What patients might or might not have agreed to, if properly informed, is beside the point.

In concluding the analysis of law's doctrine of informed consent, it should be noted that the judicial process serves two distinct but interrelated functions: the resolution of concrete disputes and the articulation of general norms. The latter involves more than the elaboration of precedent to guide future dispute resolutions. Justice Cardozo said it well: "As a system of case law develops, the sordid controversies of litigants are the stuff out of which great and shining truths will ultimately be shaped. The accidental and the transitory will yield the essential and the permanent."[35]

Yet if one wishes to discover the "great and shining truths" emerging from the doctrine of informed consent, one must look not only to what the courts said but also to what they did. A reading of the informed consent cases makes it clear that while the judges began by quite consciously stating norms, they quickly deviated from them. To be sure, 'matters of policy, rules of evidence, and the substantive law of torts and medical malpractice may have dictated such deviations. Invoking these limits, however, cannot be the end of the inquiry; for what law did not do in support of its rhetorical pronouncements must also be brought to light, exposed, and examined. Thus the reader should now pause and reflect on whether the informed consent doctrine is in practice consistent with the idea of liberty, consent, and self-determination. Whether other objectives of tort law made compromise and deviation necessary is a separate question. If they required compromise and deviation so be it. At the same time let it be acknowledged that competing claims have given short shrift to patients' right to self-determination, however much first espoused in seductive phrases.

The Retreat from Disclosure and Consent

The law of informed consent has undergone little analytic development since *Canterbury*. Except for *Scott v. Bradford*,[36] a case referred to earlier, no decisions have expanded a patient's legal protection for freedom of choice. Instead, a number of courts have gone to considerable length to reassert their faith in the capacity of doctors to set adequate disclosure standards. Already in *Collins v Meeker*,[37] decided a few years after *Natanson*, the Kansas court felt obliged to emphasize that its *Natanson* decision applied only when a physician had made "no disclosure whatever" and "that where actual disclosures have been made and are ascertainable, then expert medical testimony is required to establish that the disclosures made did not accord to those which reasonable medical practitioners would divulge under the same or like circumstances." And if not courts, then juries also asserted their faith in doctors' practices. On retrial *Canterbury* was reversed in favor of Dr. Spence.[38] A number of other celebrated cases, like *Cobbs v. Grant* (1972),[39] had similar outcomes.

In a 1976 opinion, the Supreme Court of Virginia explicitly rejected *Canterbury*: "[T]he better rule, which we now adopt, is to require a patient-plaintiff to show by qualified medical experts whether and to what extent information should be disclosed by the physician to his patient."[40] The Supreme Judicial Court of Maine adopted a similar rule in 1980.[41] In 1976, the Supreme Court of Georgia went further and held that "the 'informed consent doctrine' is not a viable principle of law in this state."[42] In *Malloy v. Shanahan* (1980),[43] the Superior Court of Pennsylvania was confronted with the question of whether Dr. Shanahan had been obligated to secure Mrs. Malloy's informed consent for treating her over a prolonged period of time with a potentially dangerous drug. The court ruled that "[s]uch informed consent is required of patient, absent an emergency, prior to a *surgical* operation. However, this has not been extended to therapeutic treatment."

In a dissenting opinion written in 1975, Justice Hanssen of the Supreme Court of Wisconsin summed up the sentiments of a great many judges, including those who had embraced the "informed consent" doctrine: "The writer has more confidence in the standards of the professional group involved than in court or jury deciding what disclosures need or ought be made to a patient facing the surgeon's scalpel. Children play at the game of being a doctor, but judges and juries ought not to."[44]

By-and-large, legislatures have echoed such retreats in their statutory enactments. Prior to 1974, the doctrine of informed consent had developed almost entirely within the common law. Yet, between 1975 and 1977, primarily in response to the medical malpractice "crisis," 24 states enacted informed consent legislation.[45] The states differed in their approaches to the problem of informed consent, but the common underlying objective generally was to blunt any rights to self-determination already granted patients by the courts. A few states, like Pennsylvania and Washington, did require that the sufficiency of disclosure be measured against the patient's need for information.[46] Many more states, however, expressly stated that compliance with customary disclosure practices of similarly situated practitioners was sufficient.[47]

Other states abandoned both the professional and the patient standards of disclosure altogether. The legislatures of both Iowa and Louisiana decided that patients needed to be informed only of the risks of "death, brain damage, quadriplegia, paraplegia, the loss or loss of function of any organ or limb, [or] disfiguring scars"[48] involved in proposed procedures.

The general intent of most legislative provisions was to protect physicians and to limit disclosure to the bare minimum. Indeed, most of these enactments erased the modest advances in patients' rights to self-determination made by earlier court rulings.

Summing up

The legal life of "informed consent," if quality of human life is measured not merely by improvements in physical custody but also by advancement of liberty, was over almost as soon as it was born. Except for the hybrid negligence law promulgated in a handful of jurisdictions and the more generally espoused dicta about "self-determination" and "freedom of choice," this is substantially true. Judges toyed briefly with the idea of patients' right to self-determination and largely cast it aside.

When the first informed consent cases came before the courts, alleging that patients had been inadequately informed by doctors and that therefore their right to self-determination had been compromised, a few judges, like Bray and Schroeder, became aware that something had gone awry in the physician-patient decision making process. They seemed to appreciate that patients were more at the mercy of physicians' unilateral interventions than courts had been accustomed to tolerate in other interactions between citizens and authorities. These judges seized on the remedy of expanding physicians' disclosure duties.

Judicial pronouncements calling for the revelation of "any facts [necessary to] an intelligent consent"[49] confronted courts with the staggering assignment of specifying what these facts were. They would have had to address complicated questions involving sophisticated inquiry: What are the risks and benefits of the proposed treatment and of no treatment? Which ones did physicians have to be aware of? How much are they required to know about them? Which ones are they required to disclose? The courts were largely unwilling and unprepared to undertake this task. Instead, they retreated to the time-honored professional standard of care, which resurfaced in disguised form even in jurisdictions that had adopted the new legal rule of disclosure.

Moreover, courts' all too single-minded emphasis on risk disclosures made the objective of giving patients a greater voice in medical decision making well-nigh unattainable. For such disclosures do little to expand opportunities for meaningful consent, particularly in surrender-prone medical settings, in which a proposed treatment is zealously advocated despite its risks. Treatment decisions are extremely complex and require a more sustained dialogue, one in which patients are viewed as participants in medical decisions affecting their lives. This is not the view of most physicians, who believe instead that patients are too ignorant to make decisions on their own behalf, that disclosure increases patients' fears and reinforces ''foolish'' decisions, and that informing them about the uncertainties of medical interventions in many instances seriously undermines faith so essential to the success of therapy. Therefore, physicians asserted that they must be the ultimate decision makers. Judges did not probe these contentions in depth but were persuaded to refrain from interfering significantly with traditional medical practices.

I have not modified my earlier assessment of law's informed consent vision:

> [T]he law of informed consent is substantially mythic and fairy tale-like as far as advancing patients' rights to self-decisionmaking is concerned. It conveys in its dicta about such rights a fairy tale-like optimism about human capacities for ''intelligent'' choice and for being respectful of other persons' choices; yet in its implementation of dicta, it conveys a mythic pessimism of human capacities to be choice-makers. The resulting tensions have had a significant impact on the law of informed consent which only has made a bow toward a commitment to patients' self-determination, perhaps in an attempt to resolve these tensions by a belief that it is ''less important that this commitment be total than that we believe it to be there.''[50]

Whether fairy tale and myth can and should be reconciled more satisfactorily with reality remains to be seen. If judges contemplate such a reconciliation, they must acquire first a more profound understanding and appreciation of medicine's vision of patients and professional practice, of the capacities of physicians and patients for autonomous choice, and of the limits of professional knowledge. Such understanding cannot readily be acquired in courts of law, during disputes in which inquiry is generally constrained by claims and counter-claims that seek to assure victory for one side.

The call to liberty, embedded in the doctrine of informed consent, has only created an atmosphere in which freedom has the potential to survive and grow. The doctrine has not as yet provided a meaningful blueprint for implementing patient self-determination. The message of this chapter is this: Those committed to greater patient self-determination can, if they look hard enough, find inspiration in the common law of informed consent, and so can those, and more easily, who seek to perpetuate medical paternalism. Those who look for evidence of committed implementation will be sadly disappointed. The legal vision of informed consent, based on *self-determination*, is still largely a mirage. Yet a mirage, since it not only deceives but also can sustain hope, is better than no vision at all.

Greater patient participation in the disclosure and consent process requires an exploration of the complex caretaking and being-taken-care-of interactions that develop between physicians and their patients. Appeals to "patient self-determination" and "physician discretion" alone do not adequately protect the participants in the medical decision-making process. Such phrases focus too much on what goes on inside the actors' separate minds and not on what should go on between them. Decision making in medicine, in order to safeguard the autonomy of both parties, must become a joint undertaking that depends more on the nature and quality of the entire give-and-take process than on whether a particular disclosure has or has not been made. Translating the ingredients of this process into useful legal and medical prescriptions that respect patients' wishes to maintain and surrender autonomy, as well as physicians' unending struggles with omnipotence and impotence in the light of medical uncertainty, is a difficult task and has not been pursued in any depth.

In the succeeding chapters I shall address many of these problems. I shall begin with the problem of professional authority and the question: Must patients blindly trust doctors' authority? Traditionally physicians have given an affirmative answer to this question; they have deemed joint decision making both unworkable and irrelevant: unworkable because medicine's esoteric knowledge creates insurmountable barriers to meaningful conversation, irrelevant because doctor's altruism provides sufficient protection to patients' interests. We now must scrutinize this authority and its justifications.

IV

Sharing Authority: The Willingness to Trust

P ATIENT PARTICIPATION in decision making will not easily
become a reality. Physicians' apprehension of, and resistance to, breaking with their millenia-long tradition of solitary decision making express not only their understandable reluctance to depart from familiar practices but also their concern
that joint decision making will bring to the public's and patients'
attention vexing problems about the state of the art and science
of medicine. Doctors believe that such problems should not be
discussed with lay persons; that a better appreciation of the uncertainty of medical knowledge will only make patients anxious
and confused.

Thus, the idea of sharing the burdens of decision with patients will create new tensions; it will also bring to the surface old
tensions that solitary decision making has obscured. They need
to be better understood and resolved before informed consent
can become more than a deceptive slogan. I have identified three
such tensions and their analysis is the subject matter of this and
the next three chapters.

The first tension is one of *authority*. Physicians throughout history have maintained that patients' needs are best served by following doctors' orders. Yet, the idea of informed consent demands joint decision making between physician and patient, a sharing of authority. Thus the question must be posed: Should either physician, patient, or both decide?

The second tension is one of *autonomy*. Meaningful decision making implies that both parties have the capacity to make choices. This notion is opposed by ancient medical beliefs that patients, by virtue of being ill, are more like children than adults and that therefore their capacity for choice is fatally impaired. Thus the question must be posed: Can anyone but a physician decide?

The third tension is one of *uncertainty*. Meaningful decision making requires that both parties have sufficient knowledge that can be imparted and understood. Medicine's vast ignorance about the etiology and treatment of disease places difficult, and at times insurmountable, burdens on physicians both to sort out for themselves knowledge from ignorance and to communicate in a comprehensible fashion their certainties and uncertainties to patients. Thus the question must be posed: How can anyone, either physician or patient, make an informed decision?

In this chapter I shall address the first tension—authority. In *Two Concepts of Liberty*, Isaiah Berlin advanced the intriguing argument that human beings complain less about a lack of liberty than about "being ignored, or patronized, or being taken too much for granted":

> The lack of freedom about which men or groups complain amounts, as often as not, to the lack of proper recognition. . . . What I may seek to avoid is simply being ignored, or patronized, or despised, or being taken too much for granted—in short, not being treated as an individual, having my uniqueness insufficiently recognized, being classed as a member of some featureless amalgam, a statistical unit without identifiable, specifically human features and purposes of my own. This is the degradation that I am fighting against—not equality of legal rights, nor liberty. . . . I desire to be understood and recognized. [W]hat I demand is an alteration of the attitude towards me of those whose opinions and behaviour help to determine my own image of myself. . . . What [I want] is simply recognition. . . .
>
> The desire for recognition is a desire . . . for union, closer understanding, integration of interests, a life of common dependence and common sacrifice. . . .[1]

Berlin's vivid depictions of human desires for recognition of their individuality, "common dependence," and equality in their interactions with one another capture an essential human striving. To recognize others fully requires not only an appreciation of their limitations but their capacities as well. Physicians have shown a keen sensitivity to patients' decision-making limitations but considerable insensitivity to their capacities to decide.

To be sure, the helplessness, anxieties, and dependence that illness engenders often makes patients appear to be less like adults with "specifically human features and purposes of [their] own" and more like children who can "be patronized [or] taken too much for granted." But instead of seeking to learn whether patients' childlikeness can be reversed, physicians have reinforced manifestations of incompetence by interacting with patients as if they were only children and not also adults. Indeed, doctors' ingrained beliefs that patients are unequal partners in the medical decision-making process have made such inquiries irrelevant. The insistence on authority has stifled any serious explorations of whether physicians and their patients could interact with one another on the basis of greater equality. Thus the idea of informed consent—of mutual decision making—remains severely compromised.

The Ideology of Professionalism

Physicians' demand for authority has received powerful reinforcement from academic scholars, particularly sociologists, who have constructed an ideology of professionalism that echoed physicians' authoritarian views of medical practice. At the heart of this ideology was an attempt to base the need for professional authority on distinctive characteristics of professions that made granting them such authority both necessary and safe from abuse. Everett C. Hughes wrote: "Professionals *profess*. They profess to know better than their clients. [They] ask to be trusted. The client is not a true judge of the value of the service he receives. . . . He must trust [doctors'] judgment and skill."[2] Similarly, Talcott Parsons, though speaking occasionally of the need for "mutuality of trust" and a "collegial" relationship between doctors and patients, also cautioned that "there must be a built-in institutionalized superiority of the professional roles."[3]

Sociologists of medicine have singled out two criteria as central to the definition of a profession: the possession of esoteric and abstract knowledge and freedom from lay control. These criteria deserve careful scrutiny. Since they are both normative and descriptive, they are flawed from the outset; since they are also influenced by self-interested and propagandistic professional motives, they are even more suspect. As Oliver Garceau observed, the only common factor in any definition of a profession is its "eulogistic terminology. . . . It apparently having been impossible to express [what a profession is] in neutral words," unless one wanted "to discredit the idea altogether."[4]

The other frequently noted criteria of a profession are derivative of the two already cited: prolonged training, a code of ethics more stringent than legal standards, concern with important, though practical, affairs of mankind, and an esteemed place in society.[5] A closer scrutiny of the two major criteria—esoteric knowledge and freedom from lay control—suggests that freedom from lay control is also a derivative characteristic of a definition of a profession. As Becker has put it, the cornerstone of the symbol of professionalism is that "[p]rofessions . . . are occupations which possess a monopoly of some esoteric and difficult body of knowledge. [It] consists not of technical skills and the fruits of practical experience but, rather, of abstract principles arrived at by scientific research and logical analysis. This knowledge cannot be applied routinely but must be applied wisely and judiciously to each case."[6] It is the "esoteric character of professional knowledge" that looms large in the demand for freedom from lay control. Without the former, the latter may be more difficult to defend.

Physicians' claim to esoteric knowledge compellingly supported their insistence on complete authority over their patients' medical needs. Parsons put this connection starkly when he concluded that "the physician is a technically competent person whose competence and specific judgments and measures cannot be competently judged by the layman. The latter must [take doctor's] judgments and measures on 'authority'."[7]

In order to buttress the claim to esoteric knowledge, so important for maintaining total control, physicians improved their standards by instituting stringent entrance requirements and extending training to maximal possible lengths. These and other strategies improved the quality of medical practice. They were also designed to impress on the public that the mastery of the mysteries of the profession is difficult and that professional knowledge can only be professed, understood, and applied by the initiated. From these assertions it was only a small step to claiming that physicians must have total control over their professional affairs and that patients must follow doctors' orders.

Granting professionals such sweeping powers, however, is dangerous for one obvious reason: the human proclivity to abuse power. To allay such fears, doctors have emphasized the protection provided by their abiding commitment to altruism, or their "collectivity (service) orientation,"[8] as sociologists have called it. Therefore, physicians have asserted that both the body politic and patients could indeed trust them. From an institutional perspective, doctors have pointed to the protection provided by the profession's ethical code and its control over individual physicians' practices. From an interpersonal perspective Parsons echoed physicians' views about the need for patients' trust when he wrote:

> [T]he patient is expected to "have confidence" in his physician, and if this confidence breaks down, to seek another physician. This may be interpreted to mean that the relationship is expected to be one of mutual "trust," of the belief that the physician is trying his best to help the patient and that conversely the patient is "cooperating" with him to the best of his ability. [T]he doctor-patient relationship has to be one involving an element of authority—we often speak of "doctor's orders."[9]

Note the quick shift from "mutual trust" to "authority."

The dual criteria of esoteric knowledge and altruism loom large in the ideology of professionalism. In fact, altruism seems to be essential to its definition; it has been employed to distinguish professions from most other groups—for example, those engaged in commerce—whose interests are deemed to be self-serving rather than altruistic. Both criteria have served well the demand for freedom from lay control: The possession of esoteric knowledge required professional authority, and altruism protected patients from any abuse of such authority.* If one be-

---

*To be sure, freedom from lay control is descriptively an important criterion of professions as they exist today; conceptually, however, it is based on the notion that esoteric knowledge requires such freedom and that altruism sufficiently safeguards patients' welfare.

lieves, as I do, that neither claim is true, the case for freedom from lay control loses much of its force in a democratic society that in principle is opposed to granting unnecessary authority to any group, particularly when such authority impinges on citizens' rights to make decisions that are most intimate and personal in nature.

Thus, in the following examination of the justifications for professional authority, freedom from lay control is not considered an essential criterion for professionalism. The possession of esoteric knowledge and altruistic commitment, however, convey something essential about professional practices and must be analyzed further. If they can survive the test of analysis, they may justify granting professionals special authority and considerable freedom from lay control.

The Story of Iphigenia

A story of an encounter with an attractive, then 21-year-old, single woman whom I first met at a panel discussion on the treatment of breast cancer, may facilitate the analysis of the problems posed by medical authority and the demand for trust in physicians that esoteric knowledge supposedly requires and altruism makes secure. I shall call the young woman Iphigenia Jones. Giving her a most common surname and a most uncommon first name—except for those familiar with Greek mythology—underscores both the frequency of the event and the rarity of what ultimately transpired, including the fact that, like her Greek sister, her sacrifice too was barely averted.[10] Some time before the panel discussion she had discovered a lump in her breast. Biopsy revealed a malignant lesion. She agreed to a mastectomy, with the extent of the surgery to be determined by what her doctor would discover during the operation. Her surgeon, who participated in the panel discussion, related to the audience his increasing doubts, as the morning of the surgery drew closer, about whether to proceed without first disclosing to Iphigenia the availability of alternative treatments, particularly radiation therapy. He had not spoken to her about alternatives because he firmly believed that surgery was the best treatment for her and that all alternatives were inferior.

Only his misgivings about having to perform such a mutilating procedure on a person that young and attractive led him to consider telling her about alternative treatments, even though such therapies were employed by other physicians at his own medical center. On the evening prior to the operation, his concerns about having remained silent, concerns that he did not fully understand, became so insistent that he returned to the hospital. He told her that, although he believed surgery to be without question the treatment of choice, alternative treatments existed and that he wished to acquaint her with them if she so desired. He added that he was not sure whether he was doing the right thing in discussing such matters with her, but he felt compelled to confide in her. Pascal had put it well: "The heart has its reasons which reason knows nothing of."[11]

They talked for a long time. Iphigenia decided that very night to postpone surgery for a few days, to consult other doctors, and then to make a choice. Eventually she opted for a lumpectomy (excision limited to the tumor mass) and radiation therapy. At the panel discussion she spoke knowledgeably and intelligently about the risks she had taken, and movingly about her impending marriage, especially her great joy over now being able to begin life with her beloved physically unscarred.

The discussion from the floor was heated and rife with controversy. Physicians defended their favorite therapies and questioned, if not attacked, other therapeutic approaches to the treatment of breast cancer. They were almost completely united on only one proposition: "It is irrational to allow patients to make these decisions." Despite Iphigenia's testimony, some asked, though the questions suggested the answer: "If doctors have such trouble deciding which treatment is best, how can patients decide? Are not patients' interests better served by trusting submission to their doctors' authority?" The physicians did not clarify the one crucial word, "best," and the senses in which they employed it.

Iphigenia's story illustrates physicians' doubts about inviting patients' participation in a decision that will deeply and irrevocably affect future welfare in very personal ways. From doctors' point of view, since patients cannot be trusted to comprehend medicine's esoteric knowledge sufficiently well, such an invitation does not make sense. Doctors believe that patients are protected far better if they trust their doctors' authority and have confidence in their altruistic dedication. Before exploring the problems of altruism and trust, I must comment briefly on the problem of esoteric knowledge, a topic that will be examined in detail in Chapter VII. What I shall say here about esoteric knowledge will not do justice to its complexity, yet it is important that I do so in order to lay the necessary foundation for the analysis of altruism and trust.

All professions possess esoteric knowledge that, in its totality, is difficult to learn, understand, and master. Indeed, the complexity of professional knowledge commands the laity to listen carefully to experts. It does not necessarily suggest, however, that this knowledge cannot be communicated to, or understood by, patients. Nor does it suggest that professionals should decide how to proceed without consulting patients, particularly if alternatives are available and treatment is beset by much uncertainty. These considerations become even more relevant if it is also correct, as I believe it is, that physicians have during this century acquired a greater capacity than they had heretofore to make distinctions between what they know, do not know, and what is as yet unknowable; that they have acquired the capacity, paradoxical as it may sound, to talk more knowledgeably about their ignorance.

The extent to which patients can understand medical knowledge is at least an open question. Physicians have had too little experience communicating their esoteric knowledge to patients to permit any conclusive answers. Beyond assertions that patients in order to understand must be given a minicourse in medicine, the literature has not seriously addressed the question: Is esoteric knowledge a serious handicap to disclosure and consent, when an effort is made to explain it? Nor have other more specific questions been asked: Which aspects of their esoteric knowledge can physicians convey and interpret to patients? When is that information sufficient to enable patients to participate in medical decision making and when might it be misleading, and why? Which aspects of a decision turn on possessing technical knowledge?

Surely, to return to Iphigenia, there is much about the accumulated knowledge of breast cancer and its treatment that is difficult to master. Many physicians avoid informing themselves about the medical controversies surrounding its treatment even though a better mastery would help them and their patients to be clearer about what is known, unknown, and conjectural. Thus the problem of esoteric knowledge is not only a patient's problem but, to begin with, a doctor's problem. A great many small, but very significant, facts about the consequences of one treatment over another are known and available. The controversies that surround the various approaches to the treatment of breast cancer can be acknowledged and explicated. It is no longer as difficult as it once was to sit down with patients and discuss the advantages and disadvantages of different treatment approaches. At least significantly more can be explained than is the general custom, and doing that would improve the climate of physician-patient decision making.

Moreover, the esoteric knowledge excuse has been employed sweepingly in order to keep silent about the simplest as well as the most complicated medical interventions. Iphigenia, about this I have few doubts, learned a great deal about the treatment of breast cancer and the consequences of whatever therapy she would finally select. Her experience alone should begin to cast doubt on the categorical assertion that any given patient is unable to sort out with her doctors which treatment suits *her* needs best. The consequences to Iphigenia of either a mastectomy, perhaps a radical one, or a lumpectomy, with or without radiation treatment, were fateful. All were treatment modalities that physicians at the hospital to which she had trustingly come were prepared to advocate as appropriate interventions. Would silence about their availability have been a preferred alternative? Should Iphigenia have placed complete trust in her surgeon's dedication to her welfare and let him decide on her behalf?

Altruism

It has frequently been asserted that physicians' altruism is safeguarded by the ancient command of *"primum non nocere*—above all, do no harm."[12] I do not wish to question physicians' commitment to giving technically good care and to not making matters worse. Professional training indeed has sought to prepare doctors for this task. Such commitments are enshrined in the Hippocratic Oath: "I will . . . abstain from whatever is deleterious and mischievous."[13] Yet the Oath continues, "I will follow that system of regimen which, according to *my* ability and judgment, I consider for the benefit of my patients. . . ." Later it goes on to say, "into whatever houses I enter, I will go into them for the benefit of the sick, and will abstain from every voluntary act of mischief and corruption. . . ."

The implications of this language are far-reaching. Note the initial emphasis on the selection of a regimen according to "my ability and judgment . . ." which is then modified by "[abstaining] from whatever is deleterious and mischievous," and by doing only what "I consider for the benefit of my patients." Two obligations bearing on patients' trust are confounded here. It is one thing to trust physicians' promise to diagnose, to treat, and not to make matters worse unnecessarily. It is quite another to trust them to know what is for their patients' benefit, in the many senses of this word, when choices are available which can make matters both better and worse.

Indeed, the original Greek version of *primum non nocere* recognized this problem. It commanded not, as does its Latin adaptation, "above all, do no harm," but rather "in the diseases we must seek two (facts): to be useful or not to damage."[14] When cure can reasonably be expected, the Greek version can be easily followed. Problems arise, however, when treatment cannot promise cure but often can only control disease, as is true for breast cancer and many other medical conditions, and when, in addition, all treatments often also inflict damage, of varying kinds and degrees. How can one both "be useful" and "not damage" in such cases? The answer cannot be reached on the basis of medical judgment alone. The blessings and curses of scientific medicine's great technological advances have greatly increased the options available to patients, but since each option entails its own significant benefits *and* risks, the horse-and-buggy notion of trust that physicians will be useful but not damage has become outmoded. The weighing of benefit and harm, which are intertwined and dependent on individual preferences, can only be carried out by patients with the assistance of their physicians. It cannot be assigned solely to physicians, no matter how pure their altruistic intent.

Thus, the most abiding adherence to professional altruism or to doctors' sacred Oath, could not provide sufficient guidance about which treatment was ultimately in Iphigenia's best interest. This undeniable truth emerged in the discussion of her case when surgeons, chemotherapists and radiation therapists seemed so convinced of the superiority of *their* treatments over those of all others. Whom should she have trusted about choice of treatment? She could only trust, and this was true in her case, that she had a most competently trained and dedicated physician, but no more and no less. She could not trust, and it almost proved true in her case, that her doctor would be honest with her and point out to her that his views were just that: *his* views.

Altruism, to the extent it exists, can only promise that doctors will try to place their patients' medical needs over their own personal needs. Even such a promise is extraordinarily difficult to fulfill in today's medical world which places such high value on economic rewards. Yet, even in the absence of any self-serving motivations, altruism cannot promise that, without conversation, physicians will know what patients' needs are or that, without conversation, patients will know in what differing ways doctors can meet their needs.

To be effectively practiced, altruism requires, as Cyrano de Bergerac appreciated so well, knowledge of his friend Christian's needs, hopes, and wishes. Cyrano knew them and on that ground could be excused for acting without asking Christian's permission. Physicians generally do not know patients' needs, although they often think they do. They need to obtain permission. Altruism cannot demand dumb trust. What was in Iphigenia's best interest could only be discovered by conversing with her, yet the doctors who discussed her case thought this was not an appropriate inquiry. Since chance determined the first choice she made of a physician, should chance have decided Iphigenia's fate? Does trust command silence?

Trust

Let me begin the analysis of trust by questioning what physicians mean when they ask patients like Iphigenia to trust them. What do they ask of her?

To trust that the treatment her physician thought best is indeed the best one for her?

To trust that her physician has adequately considered all the different senses of "best," especially the non-technical ones, before arriving at a judgment of "best"?

To trust medicine that a best treatment actually exists?

To trust that her physician can and will take the time to explain matters to her?

To trust her physician, if he discusses with her all reasonable alternative treatments, that he will do so without exerting undue pressure to choose one treatment over another?

To trust her physician to be well-informed about all available treatment modalities and to weigh and sort out all reasonable scientific, professional, and personal motivations that might influence his selecting one treatment over another?

To trust her physician that he deems her competent to contribute to the decisions that need to be made?

To trust that her physician has learned not only the language of giving comfort and orders but also of the give-and-take so necessary for joint decision making?

I could go on, but I hope that these questions sufficiently demonstrate our collective ignorance about the nature and scope of the trust that should govern interactions between physicians and patients.

Medical decision making is complex. It is influenced by many factors; for example, doctors' education, choice of specialty, scientific convictions, and economic needs. For now I only wish to focus on the problem of value judgments. As Iphigenia's story demonstrates, treatment decisions involve a combination of medical, emotional, aesthetic, religious, philosophical, social, interpersonal, and personal value judgments. Just as patients bring different values to bear on their ultimate choice, so do physicians, although doctors' value judgments are often obscured by their homogenizing all values under the single rubric of medical judgment. Indeed, one medical value—longevity—has implicitly dominated the discussion of the proper treatment of many diseases, including breast cancer, and obliterated the consideration of all other values.

The question of which judgments are purely medical ones and which are not has not received the discriminating attention it deserves. In Iphigenia's case, her surgeon was ultimately influenced by a non-medical factor, her youth, to pause and discuss her treatment with her. Eventually she too was influenced by a non-medical factor that only she could evaluate. Even if radiation treatment created a greater risk of breast cancer recurrence, she preferred to take it in order to avoid mutilation and to begin married life intact, the way she always dreamed it would turn out to be. Can anyone make such fateful decisions for another person? Listen to what a distinguished surgeon had to say about the treatment of breast cancer around the time when Iphigenia faced her decision:

> We will not revert to the regimens of partial mastectomy plus radiation therapy until *we* are satisfied that there is a reasonable probability that this form of treatment will provide a comparable length and quality of survival for those so treated. [We need controlled studies.] Such controlled studies may well *sacrifice* a generation of women but scientifically it does have merit.[15]

This doctor's words hauntingly recall Iphigenia's Greek sister. The altars of science also are presided over by gods who at times demand human sacrifice.

The need for controlled studies, though only with women's consent, is not in question. We must ask, however, whether a doctor can ask a patient to undergo radical surgery without first knowing whether the probability of a 10- to 20-year survival with radical surgery, figures that look so attractive in medical journals, means more to her than the statistical probability of a somewhat reduced life span if she chooses a less mutilating treatment. Professional altruism, so powerfully influenced by an ethical obligation to extend life at all cost—an obligation that doctors and not necessarily patients have imposed on themselves—can cruelly deceive. This, I believe, is self-evident. It should be equally self-evident that only trust in patients' capacities to sort out these issues can lead to an appropriate decision.

The superior medical knowledge that professionals possess is not the issue, but whether patients should trust physicians to decide the ultimate question of how to proceed. Eliot Freidson has addressed this problem in the general context of professional versus lay competence and authority:

> [W]e can all agree that how a road is to be built is a technical question best handled by engineers and other experts. But whether a road *should* be built at all, and *where* it should be located are not wholly esoteric technical questions. There are certainly technical considerations which must be taken into account in *evaluating* whether and where a road should be built, but engineering science contains no special expertise to allow it to decide whether a road is "necessary" and what route "must" be taken. . . . Where laymen

are excluded from such evaluation, true expertise is not at issue but rather the social and political power of the expert.[16]

In Iphigenia's case, *how* to perform surgery or administer radiation were questions for the experts. *Whether* to choose one or the other or some other treatment or no treatment was a decision that required her input as well. Freidson has said it well: "[W]hen decisions are at bottom moral or evaluative rather than substantive, laymen have as much if not more to contribute to them than have experts. This assumption reflects the substance of equality in a free society, equality not of ability, knowledge, or means, but moral equality."

Like all professionals, physicians have tried to justify their preference for trust in silence rather than in conversation on another dangerous belief: that physicians and patients have an identity of interest in medical matters. In this view, no conflict exists between them; one can decide for the other. Such contentions may have merit for the rare situations in which only one treatment reasonably promises an agreed-upon favorable result. For most medical maladies this is not the case, and the intervention that is chosen may affect a patient's subsequent state of well-being in significant ways.

The objectives of health and cure that supposedly unite physician and patient in a common pursuit can rarely be fully realized. Furthermore, these objectives can be pursued in a variety of ways, each with its own risks and benefits. The physician's personal and professional ethics and experience may dictate one course; the patient's needs, wishes, priorities, motivations, and expectations may indicate another one. Thus, health turns out to be an ambiguous state about which doctors and patients may have conflicting expectations. Physicians, in not appreciating that fact and not clarifying differences in expectations, have contributed to patients' disappointments about outcome and, in turn, to the "malpractice crisis" spawned by such disappointments.

The idea that doctors know what is in their patients' interest and therefore can act on their behalf without inquiry is so patently untrue that one can only marvel at the fervor with which the notion has been defended. One reason is clear: It makes probing conversation between doctor and patient unnecessary. The idea of inevitable conflict in all interactions between doctors and patients challenges not so much doctors' altruism but the notion that doctors can be trusted to know their patients' best interests and act on their behalf without inquiry. It also challenges not necessarily the idea that doctor and patient are one against their common adversaries—physical illness and death—but its pernicious implications that doctors' ideas of how best to fight these adversaries will also be thought best by patients. Above all it challenges the virtue of silence itself. Consider Iphigenia once again. Her surgeon believed that his way was the best and the only one to pursue. Had he proceeded with the operation as originally planned, nobody would have, or should have, questioned *his* altruistic dedication to her welfare.

Moreover, had the surgeon proceeded with the operation, few would have questioned that he had done so with her informed consent. After all, he had explained to her the nature of the intervention and *its* risks and benefits. It was an intervention approved of by the majority of physicians in his community. Since *Salgo*, physicians have increasingly provided such information to patients. But would Iphigenia's consent have been an "informed consent"? Would it have been an informed consent even if the surgeon had briefly, and in passing, mentioned that other alternatives existed but were not worth bothering much about? When throughout this book I speak about the fact that informed consent in today's world is largely a charade, I do not wish to question that a significant number of physicians now inform patients about at least some of the risks of proposed interventions. I do question, however, that many physicians inform patients about treatment options to the extent to which Iphigenia deserved to be informed.

It is odd to have to justify greater patient participation in decision making. In fact the burden of justification should reside with its opponents. As Iphigenia's experience illustrates, the decision she had to make depended less on technical and more on value judgments. Had the surgeon proceeded before talking to Iphigenia again, he would have stolen, through silence, her most basic right to decide this very personal issue that would affect the rest of her life. Luckily for Iphigenia, her surgeon learned in the last minute that she wanted to deal the common enemy a different blow.

The belief that doctors can act on behalf of patients denies the existence of inevitable conflict. Physicians' and patients' sepa-

rate identities become obliterated. They collapse into one identity and one single authoritative voice emerges—the physician's.
It alone pierces the silence and gives orders, without a need to explain the art and science of medicine or the physician's personal
and professional convictions. The authority of the physician becomes virtually absolute.

The failure to acknowledge and reconcile their separateness,
however, does not engender closeness. The opposite is true. Patients feel abandoned. They hear in doctors' recommendations
not reflections of their own wishes but of their physicians' wishes
and hopes. The distrust that accompanies the relations between
doctors and patients, analogous to the distrust that Burt described for the attorney-client relationship,[17] is a consequence of
the professed identity of caring interest, as a substitute for caring
probing of the different expectations of both parties. In such an
atmosphere, in lieu of trust, physicians only evoke feelings of ab-
ject surrender in patients.

Models of Trust

Traditional professional notions of trust are based on the wrong
model. The trust relationship that doctors prefer in interactions
with their patients mirrors the one that prevailed at the first stage
of parent-child interaction. That model emphasizes the need for
trust, in the sense of basic trust, so beautifully described by Erik
Erikson, as the only viable pattern of human interaction during
the utterly dependent earliest stage of psycho-social development.[18] Interactions between mother and infant at that time of
life are entirely nonverbal. The infant experiences a mother's
care through her deeds, and not her words.

It is not surprising that this model has been instinctively embraced by physicians and patients alike. Doctors embraced it because it called for unquestioning compliance, unilateral trust,
and verbal silence. It appealed to patients, engulfed by pain and
suffering, because surrender to powerful, wise, and soothing
caretakers was strongly fostered by memories of earlier days
when a parent satisfied all discomforting bodily needs. Thus, the
regression to more childlike functioning that can result from illness becomes augmented by a patient's wish for caretaking by a
parent-physician who, as memory informs, will immediately al-

leviate all suffering. The regression is also reinforced by doctors' proclivities to view patients as helpless and incompetent children.

When I once asked a class of senior medical students: "What kind of human beings are patients?" they responded with few dissents: "Patients are children who must be taken by the hand and guided to make the decisions we think best for them." Thus the childlikeness so often displayed by patients is triggered not only by pain, fears, illness, and memories but also by how physicians view and respond to patients. The relative contributions of each party to these regressive manifestations have not been explored. They remain shrouded in mystery.

Yet patients are not infants and physicians are not parents. Conduct appropriate and necessary for the first years of life becomes inappropriate later on. Indeed, it seems strange to have to remind medical students, and physicians as well, that patients also bring to their encounters with doctors expectations derived from subsequent stages of development: to be trusted and to trust themselves, to be allowed to stand on their own feet and not to have their dependence exploited, to be talked to and listened to, to be treated as equals and not to be ruled, to have their life style treated with respect, and to be allowed to live life in their own self-willed ways. These inherent expectations oppose the regressive pull. They often do not surface—particularly in the heady first encounters with physicians, when doctors' promises can stimulate magical hopes of finally having met the perfect caretaker.

Physicians' explicit or implicit invitation and patients' wishes to return to the infant's world of basic trust, to the paradise of Genesis, are clearly impossible dreams. Once having become an adult, a return to that world is barred, if not by angels with flaming swords, then by patients' own insights, convictions, and resistances. The much lamented distrust that so frequently intrudes on physician-patient interactions is due in part to the fact that in initial encounters with patients, professionals are all too hopeful. They readily project visions of blissful infantile security, common purpose, and understanding all their patients' needs. Such visions can only cruelly deceive and lead to resentment.

I do not question the fact that trust is an essential ingredient in interactions between physicians and patients. I only wish to propose a new kind of trust, based not on Aesculapian authority and following "doctor's orders," but on the confident and trust-

ing expectation that physicians will assist patients to make their
own decisions—decisions that in the light of their medical needs
and personal history *they* deem to be in their best interests.

The new model of trust is grounded in a number of assumptions.

First, no single right decision exists for how the life of health
and illness should be lived. Medical advances have led to a proliferation of treatment options and a better understanding of their
benefits and risks. Alleviation of suffering can be accomplished
in a variety of ways and alternative choices must be explained.
Physicians alone cannot decide which treatment is best. The patient must be consulted.

Second, physicians and patients bring their own vulnerabilities to the decision-making process. Both are authors and victims
of their own individual conflicting motivations, interests, and expectations. Identity of interests cannot be presumed. It can only
be established through conversation.

Third, both parties need to relate to one another as equals
and unequals. Their equalities and inequalities complement one
another. Physicians know more about disease. Patients know
more about their own needs. Neither knows at the outset what
each can do for the other.

Fourth, all human conduct is influenced by rational and irrational expectations. These expectations can be explored and clarified, at times more readily than at others. Reason and unreason
define human beings' essence. Manifestations of the latter should
not readily and prematurely lead to presumptions of incompetence. If they did, physicians as well as patients would have to be
labeled incompetent.

The new conception of trust advanced here only expands the
idea of trust. It asks for mutual trust that extends from physician
to patient as well as from patient to physician. This trust cannot
be earned through deeds alone. It requires words as well. It relies
not only on physicians' *technical* competence but also on their
willingness to share the burden of decision making with patients
and on their *verbal* competence to do so. It is a trust that requires
physicians to trust themselves in order to trust their patients, for
to trust patients, physicians first must learn to trust themselves to
face up to and acknowledge the tragic limitations of their own
professional knowledge; their inability to impart all their insights
to all patients; and their own personal incapacities—at times

more pronounced than at others—to devote themselves fully to their patients' needs. They must also learn not to be unduly embarrassed by their personal and professional ignorance and to trust their patients to react appropriately to such acknowledgments.

These prescriptions are difficult to translate into practice. The capacities to trust and to earn trust are not easily acquired virtues. Yet, they are necessary prescriptions if disclosure and consent are ever to become meaningful guides to decision making. The practice of medicine simultaneously seeks to wrestle with a diseased body and a diseased person, and the two are always inextricably intertwined. To give both their just due and, in case of conflict, to sort out which one to give preference, makes the practice of medicine such a difficult undertaking.

Irreconcilable conflicts between physicians and patients about the appropriate treatment of the disease and of the person, I believe, will rarely arise. Instead, if mutual trust were ever to govern physician-patient relations, the silent guerilla warfare, manifested in part by the high rate of non-compliance with doctors' orders, that now pervades their unacknowledged conflictual encounters, will significantly decrease. For the sake of respect of physicians' and patients' humanity, it is important to learn whether I am right or wrong.

Summing up

The experiment of fashioning a new ideology of professionalism that is more firmly grounded in a commitment to mutual equality, in a trusting recognition of common dependence, is worth the effort. This new ideology asserts that both physicians and patients "profess." Only after physicians have professed their esoteric professional knowledge and patients their esoteric personal knowledge, and both have confessed (another meaning of profess) to what they can do and what they expect, can a mutually satisfactory recommendation emerge. My prescription assumes that physicians and patients have the capacity to converse meaningfully with one another. I now turn to an exploration of this assumption.

V

Respecting Autonomy: The Struggle over Rights and Capacities

I N RECENT CENTURIES, the belief that persons have a right to individual self-determination has captured the imagination of the Western world. This right has been asserted on many grounds—political, philosophical, religious, moral, and legal. It also rests on the notion that human beings have the capacity to chart their own course of action in accordance with a plan they themselves have chosen.

The idea that a similar right should be accorded to patients has surfaced largely, and surely more insistently, during the last few decades. That the call for patients' right to self-determination has engendered a bitter controversy is not surprising once one appreciates that patient self-determination is an idea alien to medicine. Since physicians have generally maintained that patients do not have the *capacity* to participate in decision making, patients' "autonomy" was not a concept inscribed in medicine's vocabulary. Thus the contemporary debate over patient self-determination has been fought out over two issues that require separate consideration: rights and capacities. The proponents of patient participation in decision making have marshalled various theories of autonomy—moral autonomy, civil autonomy, and autonomy of the will—in order to assert their claims. Their opponents have argued that the demand for patient choice ignores the reality of the human incapacity to make decisions when persons become patients.

The proponents' assertions have suffered from a lack of integration of abstract notions of rights with a psychological view of human beings' capacities for autonomous choice. Any claim that individuals possess certain rights, however, presupposes an inherent capacity for the exercise of such rights. Opponents of patient self-determination, on the other hand, have not developed a systematic theory of the psychology of the physician-patient relationship. They have largely based their claims on scattered clinical observations. Even their observations have suffered from not inquiring, for example, whether the observed incapacities of patients to make decisions are fundamental to and inherent in patienthood, or engendered and reinforced by extraneous factors such as physicians' conduct. If doctors' conduct makes an essential contribution to the perceived incapacities of patients as choice makers, then such incapacities may be significantly moderated by doctors' becoming more sensitive to, and nurturing of, patients' adult capacities.

In developing a foundation for patients' rights to decision making, I shall pursue three objectives: to distinguish between rights to and capacities for decision making; to develop a more systematic view of patients' psychological capacities to chart their own course of action; and to examine the implications of my view of capacities for a right to self-determination.

Definition of Terms

Let me begin with a few broad definitions that I shall refine as I go along. The right to self-determination is defined here as the right of individuals to make their own decisions without interference from others. Autonomy has often been used interchangeably with self-determination but I shall employ the concept of autonomy, or ''psychological autonomy'' as I shall call it, to denote solely the capacities of persons to exercise the right to self-determination. In my scheme, psychological autonomy speaks to persons' capacities to reflect about contemplated choices and to make choices. The extent and limits of such capacities of course vary from individual to individual, but I am not concerned here about such individual variations. I wish to focus instead on those capacities for self-determination that depend on one's views of the psychological nature of human beings. In essense psychological autonomy is a concept that "informs" the right to self-determination by explaining, refining, and pointing up human capacities and incapacities for the exercise of such a right.

I have given autonomy's root meaning—*autos* and *nomos* = self law—an unaccustomed construction, for traditionally it has emphasized different areas of rights, be they political, legal, or moral rights. I wish to emphasize, however, the psychological capacities that underlie rights, including the right to self-determination. Indeed, underlying, although generally unidentified, assumptions about human psychology have shaped decisively the views on all political, legal, and moral rights to which persons are supposedly entitled. I retain the term autonomy to call attention to the fact that traditional definitions of autonomy, and of rights as well, contain a great many psychological assumptions that have been given insufficient consideration in understanding the complexities of decision making between physicians and patients.

The pervasive psychological assumptions that underlie autonomy and the many senses in which it has been employed, emerge in Tom Beauchamp's and James Childress' definition of autonomy:

> Autonomy is a form of *personal liberty* of action where the individual determines his or her own course of *action* in accordance with a plan chosen by himself or herself. The autonomous person is one who not only *deliberates* about and *chooses* such plans but who is *capable* of acting on the basis of such deliberations. . . . A person's autonomy is his or her independence, self-reliance, and self-contained *ability* to decide. A person of diminished autonomy, by contrast, is highly dependent on others and in at least some respect *incapable* of deliberating or acting on the basis of such deliberations. . . . The most general idea of autonomy is that of being one's own person, without constraints either by another's action or by a *psychological* or *physical* limitation. The term "autonomy" is thus quite broad, for it can refer to both *the will* and *action in society*; and both internal and external constraints on action can limit autonomy.[1]

Beauchamp and Childress appreciate that the term autonomy can be used quite broadly. It speaks in the language of rights—"autonomy is a form of personal liberty"—and in the language of capacities—"the autonomous person is one . . . who is capable of acting. . . ." To encompass both notions under the same term can lead to confusion unless great care is taken. The confusion begins to creep in, for example, when Beauchamp and Childress observe that autonomy "is his or her independence, self-reliance, and self-contained ability to decide." Do these terms address rights, capacities, or both? Moreover, striking about their definition is the emphasis on psychological criteria rather than on rights.

Similarly, Robert Veatch uses autonomy as a principle defining rights when he speaks of "inalienable rights," and as a concept defining capacities when he introduces distinctions between "autonomous" persons and those who "are substantially nonautonomous, whose actions are essentially nonvoluntary."[2] I intend to make clear distinctions between rights and capacities. I also depart from Veatch and others by not drawing distinctions between persons who are either "autonomous" or whose actions are "nonvoluntary." Instead, I start from the assumption that *all* human beings' "autonomous" functioning is affected by their capacities *and* incapacities to act "voluntarily."

Principles and Human Psychology

Abstract principles tend to express generalizations about conduct that are ill-suited for application to actual cases in which human psychological capacities to exercise rights must be considered. Abstract principles, to resolve problems posed in specific clinical situations, require mediating principles. Such mediating principles do not exist. Instead, in the fields of medical ethics and bioethics, the theoretical views of Kant, Mill, and others are often invoked to give answers to clinical problems that the principles' abstract formulations cannot provide. Such principles at best can provide a "Weltanschauung" which in the course of translation to practical cases tend to become wittingly and unwittingly infiltrated by idiosyncratic personal and professional preferences and unanalyzed assumptions about human capacities.

The conclusions drawn from these principles say more about the commentators—their orientation and assumptions—than about the principles or the problems before them. If commentators, on the other hand, try to avoid that trap by relying solely on abstract principles to guide their recommendations, their answers are too general to even come close to answering the practical questions posed by specific cases.

Yet, the problem with abstract principles is not that they are devoid of psychological assumptions, but that principles are frequently formulated without making the underlying psychological assumptions explicit. A careful scrutiny of many philosophical, moral, political or legal principles reveals all kinds of hidden, albeit woefully mutilated, assumptions about human nature. Principles, therefore, can sound foreign and strange to the heart, if not to the mind.

Immanuel Kant, in restricting his conception of autonomy to capacities to reason, without reference to human beings' emotional life and their dependence on the external world, projected a vision of human nature that estranged his principle from human beings and the world in which they must live. That Kant did so deliberately and with full awareness, because he wished to isolate and abstract a single aspect of human psychology, i.e., rationality, into its pure form, is a separate matter. What matters here is that the Kantian principle of free will, since it is based on this single aspect of human psychology, makes, if applied to actual situations, demands for human conduct that human beings cannot fulfill.

Since Kant looms large in the literature on bioethics, let me say a bit more about his views. In *Groundwork of the Metaphysic of Morals*[3], he emphasized human beings' capacity for reason. He commanded man to aspire to exercising his rational will, "to [choosing] *only that* which reason independently of inclination recognizes to be practically necessary, that is, to be good." Kant's reference to "inclination," i.e., passion, indicates that he was aware that in the real world human beings are ruled by emotions as well as reason. But Kant counselled human beings not only to resist and exercise control over inclination, but he also expected them to go a long way toward obeying only those laws that they rationally found in their uncoerced self.

Listen to his categorical imperative: "Act only on that maxim through which you can at the same time will that it should be-

come universal law.'' Kant was aware of the ''subjective imperfections of the will.'' He observed that a ''perfectly good [hu-
man] will'' would collapse the distinction between human and
divine (holy) will. But he slighted this human, empiric fact in his
theorizing. At a minimum he thought it possible to narrow the
gap decisively by exhorting each person to live by his or her categorical imperative. In doing so, Kant substituted a conception of
the rational will for the divine will—the notion that through the
exercise of reason human beings would ultimately stand, if not
closer to God, at least, as expressed in Judeo-Christian liturgy,
''just somewhat lower than the angels.''

The theoretical and aspirational nature of Kant's views of human beings must be clearly kept in mind. Kant did observe that
''the principle of humanity is not borrowed from experience . . .
it is admittedly an Ideal.'' Equally kept in mind must be Kant's
awareness that the power of ''inclination'' is buried deeply in the
human psyche. Kant only hoped that ''it must be the universal
wish of every rational being to be wholly free from them.'' Instead, some commentators have intimated, claiming Kant as authority, not that human beings *ought* to be possessed of reason
alone, but that they *can* be possessed of reason alone. Such statements have made it easier to entertain the possibility of basing
disclosure and consent upon notions of ''pure'' free will.

Such interpreters of Kant not only have failed to subject
Kant's views on human nature to a critical examination, but also
have obliterated his distinctions between theoretical man and living man. Yet Kant contributed to this misunderstanding by projecting a view of human nature that endows human beings with
greater capacities for living a life of reason than is in fact the case.
Kant's view of *theoretical* man is hopelessly estranged from *real*
man. He created the impression, perhaps unintended, that human beings can, and therefore must, employ solely their innate
and developed capacities to reason in contemplating their
choices.

When he wrote that ''in the case of men . . . the will is not in
itself completely in accord with reason,'' he did not find it necessary to ask whether ''the law of his own needs'' must be given
equal status with ''reason'' to account for the lawfulness of human nature. Instead, he proceeded to define only one facet of human behavior, the capacity for reason, and to leave unconsidered
its polar opposite, man's capacity for unreason as well as the dy-

namic interrelations between reason and unreason. I believe that even in theory, autonomy must take both polar opposites into account, for human beings are not totally possessed of either alone. Human beings are subject to the influence of reason and unreason, with the relative strength of either being affected by many innate, developmental, and situational factors. Moreover, capacities for reason are impaired whenever human beings are in pain, in love, in mourning, or in the throes of biological, environmental, or social crises. Kant's theoretical conception of the nature of human beings is too neglectful of the complex interrelations between reason, emotions, and the external world; it is therefore of little relevance to practical situations. The debate over the relevance of principles to the resolution of human problems needs to encompass a new dimension and pose new questions: To what extent should principles comport with the biological, psychological, and social nature of human beings? To the extent that they do not, what is the relevance of such principles as guides to human conduct?

Self-Determination and Psychological Autonomy

I have already suggested that psychological autonomy and self-determination, although interrelated, need to be clearly distinguished. I shall use self-determination to refer only to the rights of individuals to make decisions without interference by others. At its extreme, it is an ideal construct, unattainable in human affairs, as the need for civil, criminal, and moral laws restricting certain conduct clearly indicates. Paternalism, one of self-determination's contrary siblings, is a principle on the same level of abstraction. At its extreme, it implies total surrender of decision making to the will of others. The debate about patient self-rule in physician-patient interactions has sought to pinpoint the location of the right to make decisions on the continuum between self-determination and paternalism.

Self-determination contains, as my discussion on psychological autonomy will soon make clearer, two intertwined, though separable ideas. One looks at conduct in relation to the external world, at conduct in relation to action. I call this external component of self-determination *choice*. It has also been spoken of as freedom of action. The other looks at conduct in relation to the internal world, at conduct in relation to thinking about choices by oneself and with others prior to action. I call this internal component of self-determination *reflection* or *thinking about choices.* Traditionally, discussions of self-determination have emphasized the external component. I shall argue instead that both the external and internal components deserve equal and separate consideration.

Psychological autonomy refers to the extent and limits of a person's capacities to reflect and to make choices inherent in the psychological nature of human beings. As an ideal construct, psychological autonomy refers to the capacity of persons to reflect, choose, and act with an awareness of the internal and external influences and reasons that they would wish to accept. It must be clearly kept in mind that this is an ideal definition. Choice on the basis of a complete awareness of the influences and reasons that impinge on it is never attainable, but awareness can be significantly improved through self-reflection and conversation with others.

Internal Reflection and External Choice

A number of considerations have led me to introduce distinctions between internal reflection and external choice, as well as to highlight the importance of psychological autonomy. The external-internal distinction permits the posing of two sets of fundamentally different questions about persons' capacities for psychological autonomy. One external question is: "To what extent should an individual's *choices* be respected?" Two internal questions are: "To what extent should an individual's *thinking about choices* be respected?" and "Can and should a person's capacity for reflection be enhanced through conversation?" The last question is important if I am correct in assuming that human psychological capacities for autonomy are limited, yet subject to enhancement by conversation.

In all human encounters the respect accorded to self-determination is influenced by assumptions about human beings' psychological capacities to think and to act. The only psychological assumption that the medical profession has acknowledged and endorsed is that patients under the stress of illness and as a result of ignorance about medical matters are incapable of making decisions on their own behalf. The external-internal distinction draws attention to a crucial question that challenges this assumption: If physicians were to provide patients with a meaningful opportunity for conversation, could whatever incapacities to reasoning illness engenders be moderated sufficiently for patients' choices to be treated with greater respect? It is likely that the answer would be affirmative for a significant number of patients, particularly those who do not suffer from acute illnesses. If physicians were to pay greater attention to conversation—to patients' capacities to reflect about choices—it could change their traditional attitudes toward patients' capacities to make their own decisions and, in turn, could radically transform the current state of physician-patient decision making.

The respect one wishes to accord to the internal and external components of self-determination, however, also depends upon how one weighs political, legal, and moral value preferences such as privacy, beneficence, loyalty and freedom. Looked at from this perspective, the external component also encompasses the choices individuals must be allowed to exercise to uphold these values (e.g., respect for liberty and freedom of action) and the internal component encompasses the extent of reflection and conversation that individuals should be obligated to engage in prior to acting, to respect these values. For example, respect for the great importance physicians place on beneficence and loyalty to their patients may suggest that physicians have a right and need to be informed why their patients do not choose to follow a proposed course of action so that doctors can be reasonably certain that their patients have understood their recommendations.

The internal-external distinction also permits separate consideration of the relevance of assumptions about human psychological functioning to reflection, on the one hand, and to choice, on the other. Whenever patients' right to self-determination has been discussed, the focus of discussion about psychological capacities has been on choice. The proponents of self-determination have argued that the choices of all but incompetent individuals must be honored and that the introduction of any psychological assumptions is irrelevant or even treacherous. For the most part, I share these views. Even though choices are influenced by psychological considerations, it is one thing to appreciate that fact and quite another to interfere with choice on the basis of speculations, or even evidence, about underlying psychological reasons that seemingly led a patient to make the "wrong" choice. Such psychological explanations can be found too readily and exploited too easily for purposes of over-reaching and coercion. Thus the dangers of interfering with patients' choices on psychological grounds are too great and too difficult to control. Short of substantial evidence of incompetence, choices deserve to be honored.

Reflection, however, deserves to be treated differently. Here psychological assumptions suggest that physicians and patients are under an obligation to reflect and to converse. Ignorance, misconceptions, exaggerated fears, and magical hopes about matters such as diagnostic tests and therapeutic interventions, as well as about what physicians and patients want and are able to do for one another, can decisively influence choice. The danger is great that patients' and doctors' choices will be distorted by such internally and externally engendered mistaken ideas. Thus, conversation will have to be more extensive and more searching if one believes that such distortions affect choice and that they can and must be sorted out. On the other hand, such conversation can be more limited if one holds to the belief that thought and action are based largely on a reasoned awareness by both parties of the motivations and reality factors that influence their conduct.

Finally, the separation of the internal from the external aspects of self-determination helps to focus attention on the largest, yet least examined, problem in physician-patient decision making: physicians' unquestioning acceptance of patients' affirmative responses to a proposed intervention. The right to self-determination has most extensively been discussed in relation to refusals of diagnostic and therapeutic procedures, that is, in relation to honoring "negative" choices. However important an issue, outright refusals are rare events in physician-patient encounters.

Affirmative responses deserve study in their own right. Doctors' acceptance of a mere "yes" response is often meaningless because they have no idea what it means to the patient. In addition, an all too ready acceptance of a "yes" response can constitute what Edmond Cahn has called an "engineering of consent by exploiting the condition of necessitous men."[4] Cahn identified a most troublesome flaw in physician-patient conversation: the witting and unwitting manipulation of disclosure and, in turn, of choice by trading on the ignorance and fears of scared patients. For example, this can happen in instances of "unnecessary surgery," when an elective procedure, such as a hysterectomy for fibroid tumors, is represented without qualifications as the one medically indicated to "avoid cancer." If I am correct that the process of thinking about choices can be improved, then subsequent problems of disagreement between physicians and patients over choice, or patients' outright refusals, may prove to be less disturbing than they now are. Attention to thinking about choices may either reconcile physicians' and patients' differences in expectations or clarify the differences sufficiently for both to feel more comfortable in going their separate ways.

Psychoanalytic Considerations

My views on self-determination have been shaped by psychoanalysis, particularly by the concepts of conscious-unconscious, rationality-irrationality, and primary and secondary process. A brief presentation of these concepts is offered to clarify the subsequent discussion of my views on psychological autonomy and their implications for decision making between physicians and patients. Of course, psychoanalysis is only one of many theories about human psychology and my views must be evaluated from the vantage point of my specific theoretical commitment. Whether one adheres to psychoanalytic theory or not, however, one must commit oneself to some psychological theory, for assumptions about human nature loom large in whatever views one entertains about self-determination and decision making between physicians and patients.

The pervasive influence of the unconscious on the lives of human beings has been one of psychoanalysis' most significant discoveries. After amassing extensive data on his own and his patients' symptoms, dreams, and ordinary mistakes, Sigmund Freud concluded that:

> [M]ental processes are in themselves unconscious and . . . of all mental life it is only certain individual acts and portions that are conscious. [P]sychoanalysis . . . cannot accept the identity of the conscious and the mental. It defines what is mental as processes, such as feeling, thinking, and willing, and it is obliged to maintain

that there is unconscious thinking and unapprehended willing. . . . [T]he hypothesis of there being unconscious mental processes paves the way to a decisive new orientation in the world of
science.[5]

The proposition that "there are purposes in people which can become operative without their knowing about them" raises challenging problems for traditional notions of individual autonomy,
as well as for legal, moral, philosophical, and political views
about human nature. Such views on autonomy generally seem to
assume either that human beings can readily become aware of
the significant intentions that shape their conduct or that unconscious intentions can or should be disregarded.

Psychoanalysis, on the other hand, asserts that any conception of psychological autonomy must take the unconscious into
account. If both conscious and unconscious forces affect behavior—or, as Stuart Hampshire has put it, if "the occasions on
which we have, to a greater or lesser degree, misrepresented to
ourselves what we are trying to do is much more common than
we had previously believed"[6]—then human beings are not totally
free, in the sense of being fully conscious about why they act in
certain ways. The importance psychoanalysis attributes to the
unconscious also suggests that we can become "freer" only if we
acknowledge that unconscious motivations influence the decisions we make and then explore the sources of these motivations,
or at least appreciate the influence of such hidden forces on
thought and action.

A functional definition of psychological autonomy, therefore,
must encompass unconscious purposes. It must take into account
that an ideational system can exercise motivational force without
being introspectively accessible. Yet the presence of unconscious
forces, and their impact on thought and action, are not the only
factors that must be considered in arriving at a more appropriate
concept of psychological autonomy. Attention must also be paid
to the existence of conflict between conscious and unconscious
motivations. Such conflicts generally lead to compromise formations that, once they reach consciousness, can express, for example, motivations that have less to do with one's current situation
and more with unresolved problems from earlier years. Thus
one's conscious thought or action may distort one's current
needs and desires.

A second psychoanalytic concept important for an understanding of psychological autonomy is primary and secondary process. In his biography of Freud, Ernest Jones observed that "Freud's revolutionary contribution to psychology was not so much his demonstrating the existence of an unconscious, and perhaps not even his exploration of its content, as his proposition that there are two fundamentally different kinds of mental processes, which he termed primary and secondary respectively, together with his description of them."[7] The existence of two different kinds of mental processes, each following its own laws, has profound implications for the conceptualization of psychological autonomy. I shall refer to these processes as irrationality and rationality respectively. (The two sets of terms are roughly equivalent, except that rationality-irrationality is not weighted down with the same specific meanings as primary and secondary processes, important to psychoanalysis but not to the present discussion.)

Thought and action are influenced by the simultaneous operation not only of conscious and unconscious forces but also of rational and irrational determinants. Thought and action are rarely, if ever, under the domination of either rationality or irrationality alone, and the admixture of the two differs from person to person, and for the same person under the impact of different external conditions. The mixture is also affected by the quality of the conversation between persons.

Rationality refers to the impact on thought and action of consciousness, reality needs, time perspectives, varied and subtly blended emotions, realistic expectations, necessary postponements of gratification, reflective thought prior to action, and regard for facts. Irrationality refers to the impact on thought and action of unconscious impulses and ideation, fantasies, timelessness, concreteness, unmodulated emotions, confusions of past and present realities, unattainable and infantile conceptions, and disregard of facts. Roy Schafer has made the important point that the contrasts drawn between rationality and irrationality "present ideal polar positions. Any specific behavior must be assessed . . . in terms of the particular admixture of [rationality and irrationality] in it. There are all degrees of transition."[8]

Conscious-unconscious and rational-irrational are often erroneously used interchangeably. They need to be distinguished. When I use "conscious-unconscious" I wish to convey that thought and action are simultaneously influenced by determinants of which the individual is both aware and unaware. The degree of awareness-unawareness will vary, but complete awareness is never possible: "Conscious-unconscious" refers to internal mental states, to the constant interplay of consciousness and unconsciousness on thoughts and feelings.

The terms "rational-irrational" highlight capacities for adaptation to the external world, that is, persons' conscious and unconscious efforts to reconcile their internal mental processes with the external possibilities and limitations of the world in which they live. They denote persons' abilities to take reality into account and to give some account of the conflicts between their inner and outer worlds to themselves and others. An observer's evaluation of a subject's rationality and irrationality must encompass information on how the subject perceives the external world. Since persons may perceive the world in different ways, observer and subject can differ radically on what they consider rational and irrational. This fact makes the evaluation of rational-irrational more a matter of interpersonal dynamics than is true for conscious-unconscious which depends more on how individuals react *qua* themselves. Thus, any evaluation of perceived "irrational" conduct must take into account that such a judgment may be based on differences in values, life style, and other personal matters between the two interacting parties.

Take Iphigenia as an example. It is one thing to say that her choice of radiation therapy was influenced by unconscious factors and another to say that it was, as some physicians believed, an irrational choice. Whether it was "rational," however, depends on how one balances the competing values of longevity and physical appearance. Iphigenia decided to adapt to the world in which she wished to live by opting for radiation therapy and she gave a reasonably good account of her choice. It was an irrational choice only if one assumes that she should have adapted to her world differently. Some doctors believed that she should have made a different choice, but this only proves that her and their value preferences diverged. The irrational ones were those doctors who could not entertain the idea that they and she might differ on what is rational.

Therefore an assessment of rationality-irrationality in medical decision making demands a new inquiry based not only on an understanding of patients' views in relation to their perceptions of the world but also on a scrutiny by both physicians and patients of the significance to be assigned to their respective views of the other's "irrationality" and their own "rationality." It often will turn out that positions must be reversed. For example, it may turn out that what a physician first perceived to be an expression of a patient's "irrational" behavior was based on different value preferences about the importance of longevity, quality of life, bodily invasions, or the risks a patient is willing to take for purposes of greater well-being. Neglect of such influences has often led doctors to label a patient's judgment irrational prematurely, without a sustained effort to sort out their own and their patients' reasons for choices recommended or made.

Efforts at clarification need to be conducted in the spirit of a better understanding of the context in which the "irrationalities" have arisen. Premature struggles to convince the other of his or her "irrationality" are counterproductive; they only preclude the possibility of mutual understanding.

Irrationality may be conscious or unconscious. Consciousness of a thought or action does not determine its rationality. "The rational plan," as Heinz Hartmann put it, "must [always] include the irrational as a fact."[9] Optimal ego functioning employs rational regulations and simultaneously takes into account the irrationality of other mental achievements.

Therefore, irrational thought must not be equated with pathology. It is an essential ingredient of life, as it is of the life of dreams, artistic creations, and scientific achievements. Hans Loewald has expressed all this well:

> . . . Not only do irrational forces overtake us again and again; in trying to lose them we would be lost. The id, the unconscious modes and contents of human experience, should remain available. If they are in danger of being unavailable—no matter what state of perfection our "intellect" may have reached—or if there is danger of no longer responding to them, it is our task as historical beings to resume our history making by finding a way back to them so that they may be transformed, and away from a frozen ego. . . .

*   *   *

Freud called the dynamic unconscious indestructible in comparison with the ephemeral and fragile, but infinitely precious, formations of consciousness. Where id was, there ego shall come into being. Too easily and too often ego is equated with rigid, unmodulated, and unyielding rationality. So today we are moved to add: where ego is, there id shall come into being again to renew the life of the ego and of reason.[10]

Indeed, paradoxical as it may sound, exclusion of all irrationality leads to pathology. Obsessive-compulsive personalities are living examples of this point.

Thus, in conceptualizing autonomy in terms of the simultaneous operation of rationality and irrationality, it is important to recognize that one does not necessarily speak to the healthy, and the other to the pathological, aspects of human behavior. Both activities can define normal and abnormal human psychological functioning. They work hand in hand. If either is impaired, human conduct is impaired. One is not an expression of man's "lower nature" and the other of man's "higher nature." I do not believe that these observations blunt my argument that through conversation and self-reflection the impact of the unconscious and of irrationality on thought and action can be reduced and that doing so is to the good. My observations only emphasize that before the unconscious and irrational influences on thought and action can be evaluated, they need to be identified and compared with one's views of oneself and of one's world.

The two sets of distinctions—conscious-unconscious and rational-irrational—have different implications for psychological autonomy. If I am correct in assuming that greater consciousness of the determinants that influence thought and action can enhance decision making, then attempts to achieve such an awareness through self-reflection and reflection with others become necessary for optimal decision making. On the other hand, given human beings' limited capacities for greater consciousness and the fact that unconscious thoughts may express integrated, essential, and significant wishes, beliefs, and values of the individual, unawareness does not suggest that a person has not made a "good" decision. If these statements sound paradoxical, they only attest to the fact that human psychology contains many paradoxes. Yet the paradox can be placed in better perspective: It is more of a paradox if one expects reflection to lead to total consciousness and rationality. The paradox becomes significantly reduced, however, if one only expects reflection to make it more certain that persons do not fall victims to those irrational and unconscious influences that they wish to avoid *and*, with reasonable care, can recognize.

My concerns about assuming that unconscious and irrational motivations are always inherently inferior also have practical implications. For example, unawareness cannot be taken as a justification for substituting professional judgments for those of a patient in the belief that it is in the latter's "best interest" or that a patient would have followed doctors' orders if he had only been more rational. In his lectures on *Two Concepts of Liberty*, Isaiah Berlin eloquently spoke to the danger of ignoring persons' wishes based on the notion that "they are actually aiming at what in their benighted state they consciously resist, because there exists within them an occult entity—their latent rational will, or their 'true' purpose." He continued:

> This monstrous impersonation, which consists in equating what X would choose if he were something he is not, or at least not yet, with what X actually seeks and chooses, is at the heart of all political theories of self-realization. It is one thing to say that I may be coerced for my own good which I am too blind to see; and another that if it is for my good, I am not being coerced, for I have willed it, whether I know this or not, and am free even while my poor earthly body and foolish mind bitterly reject it, and struggle against those who seek however benevolently to impose it, with the greatest desperation.[11]

These dangers to which Berlin alerted the world of rulers and citizens have been insufficiently heeded in the world of physicians and patients as well. Since Hippocratic days, physicians have asserted that their rational individual and professional commitment to the pursuit of health can be distinguished from the common irrationality of patients who, by virtue of ignorance and/or illness, may not pursue their own enlightened self-interests. Such views of patients have also led doctors to argue that patients would have agreed to the choices made for them if their real self had been in better control. Thus when doctors control choices by silence and evasions, they do not deem it to be a form of coercion. Instead, doctors believe that such conduct is guided only by their considerations of patients' own good at a moment in time when patients are too blind to see it for themselves.

Berlin despaired of the likelihood of controlling such abuses. Perhaps he gave up too easily. In time, the conflicted nature of human beings—the inevitable presence of internal and interpersonal disharmony and tension as well as the constant interplay of consciousness and unconsciousness, of rationality and irrationality—may be more fully accepted, and its influence on both rulers and the ruled, physicians and patients, acknowledged. If that were to happen, perhaps the abuses of such concern to Berlin will be better contained. If I am correct, then individual freedom should be equated neither with simply permitting patients to do what they initially desire nor with requiring them simply to make complete sense to their physicians. Instead, and above all, respect for freedom would demand respectful conversation. True freedom entails constant struggle and anguish with oneself and with others. This is the lesson of psychoanalysis and its theories about human conduct and interactions.

Implications for Physician-Patient Decision Making

In contrast to other definitions of psychological autonomy, mine is not solely "linked . . . to those higher forms of consciousness that are distinctive of human potential."[12] I reject such artificial restrictions to conduct regulated primarily by reason. Since reason and unreason always act in concert, both are facets of psychological autonomy. I now turn to the implications of my views on psychological autonomy for decision making between physicians and patients.

First, thought and action can never be brought fully under the domination of consciousness and rationality. Physicians and patients, however, can become more aware of the ever-present and pervasive impact of the unconscious and of irrationality on thought and action. An appreciation of the limits of rationality would sensitize physicians and patients to the need for subjecting their thoughts and contemplated actions to prior reflection, both alone and with one another. It would also sensitize them to the inevitable persistence, even after conversation, of lingering, nagging, and quite healthy doubts about the continuing influence of unconscious and irrational determinants on their conduct. Such an awareness, which unites physicians and patients in common vulnerabilities, can only make them more careful about apodictic judgments and more respectful of conflicting wishes and expectations.

For example, physicians would have to pay greater attention to reflection if they believed that their conduct was influenced by the same underlying unconscious and irrational determinants as that of their patients. The contrary assumption, that doctors', but not patients', contributions to any conversation are influenced largely by rational (personal and professional) considerations, has made self-reflection by physicians and even searching conversation between physicians and patients—from which *both* can learn—largely irrelevant. If physicians and patients recognized that physicians' communications are also affected by unconscious and irrational determinants, the parties' perceptions of one another and conversations between them would be decisively affected. Awareness of the irrationalities that physicians bring to decision making has been impeded by the idea that medical decision making involves largely technical-scientific issues that physicians can evaluate more rationally than patients can. Technical issues, however, as Iphigenia's story illustrates, are only one of the determinants that impinge on thinking about choices.

Second, the simultaneous domination of thought and action by rational and irrational, conscious and unconscious, determinants can be shifted in the direction of greater rationality and consciousness. At a minimum ill-considered and mistaken ideas can be clarified, uncertainties specified, fears dispelled, and the confusions of past experiences that have no relevance to the present situation untangled. Self-reflection and reflection with others can aid this process immeasurably. Thus, physicians and patients need to engage in conversation to clarify their mutual expectations to the extent possible. Most importantly, physicians must assume the primary obligation of facilitating such conversation.

Indeed, I take a further step and postulate a duty to reflection that cannot easily be waived. Asserting such a duty sounds strange. We are accustomed to recognizing a right to choice as an aspect of the right to self-determination, but a duty to reflection as a component part of the concept of autonomy is quite another matter. Yet, if my views on psychological autonomy have merit, then respect for the right to self-determination requires respect for human beings' proclivities to exercise this right in both rational and irrational ways. Doctors are obligated to facilitate patients' opportunities for reflection to prevent ill-considered rational and irrational influences on choice.

Patients, in turn, are obligated to participate in the process of thinking about choices. In arguing that both parties make every effort to facilitate reflection in order to sort out the rational and irrational expectations that eventually can converge on choice, I express a value preference for the enhancement of individual psychological autonomy. John Stuart Mill, the most celebrated and uncompromising champion of "liberty of action,"[13] anticipated my views on the need for conversation. He eloquently argued that his "principle"—that "the sole end for which mankind are warranted, individually or collectively, in interfering with the liberty of action of any of their number, is self-protection"—is misunderstood if it is interpreted to require "selfish indifference, which pretends that human beings have no business with each other's conduct in life." He most insistently asserted instead that "[c]onsiderations to aid his judgment, exhortations to strengthen his will, may be offered to him, even obtruded on him, by others." Only after such an enforced conversation must individual men and women be allowed to be "the final judge," since "they have means of knowledge [about their feelings and circumstances] immeasurably surpassing those that can be possessed by anyone else."

Thus, Mill, whose concern over human "fallibility" had a significant impact on his insistence for liberty of action, may also have instinctively appreciated that human beings' psychological functioning is fragile and can readily be compromised. Therefore he advocated invasions of privacy through exhortations and obtrusions. He may have recognized that human beings' psychological functioning needed nurture and support in the service of "freedom of action." That amount of intrusion, that degree of paternalism, he tolerated, indeed advocated. He hoped that such intrusions would be carried on with a clear recognition by both parties that the choice ultimately made, no matter how foolish or idiosyncratic, must be honored. Mill viewed this imposition of dialogue as a necessary corrective to the uncompromising demand for liberty of action. It also foreshadowed the distinctions I have introduced between internal reflection and external choice.

Mill fervently believed in man's rational nature. He observed that "on the whole [there is] a preponderance among mankind of rational opinions and rational conduct." Yet he was aware of at least one facet of man's propensity to irrationality—the pervasive need to deny fallibility. "Unfortunately for the good sense of mankind," he wrote, "the fact of their fallibility is far from carrying the weight in their practical judgment which is always allowed to it in theory; for while everyone well knows himself to be fallible, few think it necessary to take any precautions against their own fallibility.'' The existence and denial of fallibility became a crucial argument in support of conversation. ''Human beings owe to each other help to distinguish the better from the worse, and encouragement to choose the former and avoid the latter. But neither one person, nor any number of persons, is warranted in saying to another human creature of ripe years, that he shall not do with his life for his own benefit what he chooses to do with it.''

His awareness of man's irrationality, as evidenced by man's denial of fallibility alone, was sufficient reason for Mill to assert the necessity of both freedom of action and conversation. ''[Man's] errors,'' he wrote, ''are corrigible. He is capable of rectifying his mistakes, by discussion and experience. Not by experience alone. There must be discussion, to show how experience is to be interpreted.''

In my view, the right to self-determination about ultimate choices cannot be properly exercised without first attending to the processes of self-reflection and reflection with others. This holds true for patients as well as for physicians. Contrary views have paid insufficient respect not only to human proclivities for unconscious and irrational decision making but also, and more importantly, to the possibilities of bringing some of these determinants to greater awareness. Such views on autonomy and self-determination do not pay respect to ''self-defined'' individuals; instead, such views inhibit opportunities for women and men to become clearer about how they may wish to define themselves, abandoning them instead to a malignant fate. In the context of physician-patient decision making, it must be recognized that illness—including the fears and hopes it engenders, the ignorance in which it is embedded, the realistic and unrealistic expectations it mobilizes—can contribute to tilting the balance in patients and physicians further toward irrationality and choices that, on reflection, both might wish to reconsider. In short, I seek to justify the duty to reflection on the grounds of human beings' capacities to take their unconscious and irrationality more fully into account.

I am not suggesting, however, that the conversations between physicians and patients be converted into an exploration of the psychological roots of patients' and physicians' motivations and expectations. This is neither warranted nor possible. I have in

mind only a bona fide attempt by physicians and patients to explain what they wish from one another and what they can do for
and with one another, and to clarify, to the extent possible, any
misconceptions they may have of each others' wishes and expectations. In the end, irreconcilable differences may persist. If they
then realize that they must part company, at least they will do so
with a greater appreciation of their respective positions.

The third implication of my views on psychological autonomy
is that the limitations inherent in fully knowing oneself or others,
and their potential tragic implications for choice making and
choice, demand thoughtful consideration of whether and when to
interfere with patients' choices. One must determine when such
limitations justify interference with choice or thinking about
choice and whether such interferences comport with fidelity to
other values, such as respect for dignity, integrity, equality, loyalty, health, and beneficence. For example, mere acceptance of
patients' "yes" or "no" response to a proposed intervention
may not express respect for their self-determination, dignity, or
integrity. Indeed, blindly accepting either response may violate
their integrity and constitute an act of disloyalty to the person.
Either response, if accepted without question, is disrespectful of
patients' capacities for reflective thought, which might have led
to a different choice more consonant with their own wishes and
expectations. This is particularly true for a "yes" response to a
doctor's recommendations accompanied by a patient's disclaimer
of a need for information. At least for some time to come, the traditional medical climate in which patients are expected and expect to follow doctors' orders will continue to force patients to ab-
dicate decision-making responsibility for reasons that doctors
should question and put to rest. For example, on inquiry, patients may reveal their concerns about imposing on physicians'
time, their fears about annoying doctors with their questions, or
their embarrassment about not being able to ask the right questions without assistance from their doctors. These and other fears
and misconceptions need to be dispelled. A patient's waiver of
the physician's obligation to disclose and obtain the patient's
consent should be accepted only after a committed effort has
been made to explore the underlying reasons for the patient's ab-
dication of decision-making responsibility.

In opposition to such suggestions, doctors have frequently asserted that most patients wish physicians to decide for them with-

out much prior conversation, and that doctors only support the wisdom of such desires. If this assertion is true, then the demand for conversation is disrespectful of physicians' and patients' wishes. This problem deserves careful study. In a recent interview the author-surgeon Richard Selzer was asked whether he had developed a philosophy about how much a patient has a right to know. He responded:

> The patient has a right to know everything. The patient may not wish to know everything. Ever since the 1960's, we've been told that the patient must be the colleague of his doctor and that the decision-making must be shared equally by the two of them. Intellectually and philosophically I certainly do agree. Unfortunately, it doesn't quite work out that way. When I try to call the patient in on a consultation and say, "Which alternative would you prefer?" *invariably* the patient says, "What do you mean, which alternative? I want you to tell me what to do. You're the doctor." The only unspoken word is daddy; tell me what to do, daddy. When a person is desperately ill or frightened, there is a certain kind of regression that makes you want to place yourself in someone's loving care. It is the responsibility of the doctor to have the courage to make decisions for the patient, in as kind and wise a way as he can. To be a father or mother and comfort. There are, of course, strong people who want to know everything and decide everything but they are a distinct minority.[14]

It is unclear from the interview whether Selzer tries to explore patients' statements, "I want you to tell me what to do. You're the doctor," before submitting to their request. A surgeon might very well say to a patient, in response to "I want you to tell me": "Of course I shall eventually give you my recommendation, but I prefer not to do so yet. Since there are a number of alternatives available, each with its risks and benefits, I would like to hear first what your preferences are. After all it is *your* body that I intend to treat and I can do so in a variety of ways. Since you will have to live with your body for a long time to come, you must have some opinions about which consequences would be easier or more difficult for you to tolerate. Once I have a better idea of your preferences and needs, I can make a recommendation that reconciles the best that surgery has to offer with the best that you envision for yourself after I have discharged you from my care."

Surely many physicians "hear" the "unspoken word . . . daddy" too readily in patients' voices. They then proceed to take care of their patients without further inquiry, much as Dostoy-evsky's Grand Inquisitor suggested human beings wish to be dealt with:

> There are three forces, the only three forces that are able to conquer and hold captive the conscience of these weak rebels for their own happiness—these forces are: miracle, mystery and authority. . . . Is the nature of man such that he can reject a miracle and at the most fearful moments of life, the moments of his most fearful, fundamental, and agonizing . . . problems, stick to the free decision of the heart? [S]ince man is unable to carry on without a miracle, he will create new miracles for himself, miracles of his own, and will worship the miracles of the witch-doctor and the sorcery of the wise woman. . . . And men rejoiced that they were once more led like sheep and that the terrible gift [of freedom] which had brought them so much suffering had at last been lifted from their hearts. . . . Tell me. Did we not love mankind when we admitted so humbly its impotence and lovingly lightened its burden . . .?[15]

The Grand Inquisitor's views of human nature, shared by many physicians, have shaped the conversations between persons in powerful and self-fulfilling ways. There may be other unspoken messages in patients' voices, however, that ask at least for a father who appreciates that his children are not only children but also adults who wish and deserve to be heard. If doctors were to listen more to these adult voices, they might learn that more patients prefer to participate in decision making than physicians commonly believe. The task of distinguishing between patients who wish to be treated as adults or as children still needs to be undertaken.

The fourth implication of my views on psychological autonomy is that the requirement for conversation creates inevitable conflicts with the right to privacy—the right to keep one's thoughts and feelings to oneself. Thus, the imposition of an obligation to converse is disrespectful of the right to have one's initial choice, including the right not to converse, honored. Refusals to converse, however, totally obscure both patients' and doctors' understanding of how they arrived at their decision. This is particularly true when patients either decline a needed medical intervention or accept it unquestioningly. Respect for psychological autonomy becomes severely compromised when refusals or acceptances are heeded without question. Here the principle of privacy must bend to psychological autonomy. (This may turn out to be a rare Hobson's choice, for I expect that most patients, if invited by their physicians, will welcome conversation.)

Fifth, the posited obligation to converse introduces an element of paternalism into my prescription. Yet, it must also be recognized that my views about psychological autonomy and its accompanying obligations to reflect and converse seek to avoid paternalism and to strengthen patient self-determination. The obligations that I advocate are imposed on *both* parties; they do not ask for one party to submit to the other; they are grounded in mutuality; and they are dictated by a respect for human psychological functioning in the specific context of physician-patient decision making: patients' wishes to be an adult *and* a child, and doctors' wishes to treat patients more as children than as adults.

Respect for psychological autonomy requires that both parties pay caring attention to their capacities and incapacities for self-determination by supporting and enhancing their real, though precarious, endowment for reflective thought. In conversation with one another, patients may uncover mistaken notions about their diseases and their treatment that they have held for a long time or have recently acquired through misunderstanding the import of their doctors' recommendations. Physicians may uncover the fact that their unconscious preferences and biases compelled patients to yield to their recommendations even though consciously they had intended otherwise. Without conversation, individual self-determination can become compromised by condemning physicians and patients to the isolation of solitary decision making, which can only contribute to abandoning patients prematurely to an ill-considered fate.

It has been said that remonstrances against paternalism, while logically not inconsistent with concern for others, may nevertheless diminish one's concerns for others. Karl Marx said it more strongly: "the right of man to liberty is based not on the association of man with man, but on the separation of man from man. It is . . . the right of the restricted individual, withdrawn into himself."[16] While there is some truth in these statements, it must be remembered that except in the rarest of circumstances, the ultimate decision belongs to the patient who has to live with the decision. One can only try to help a patient to make *his* or *her* best choice. Both of these considerations loom large in my distinction between reflection and choice.

Summing up

This chapter highlighted the crucial significance of the concept of psychological autonomy to a better understanding of the principle of self-determination. The respect accorded to self-determination and, in turn, to disclosure and consent is affected by assumptions about human capacities for reflection and choice. If I am correct that a comprehensive definition of individual autonomy must take into account the conscious and unconscious, rational and irrational forces that shape all thoughts and actions, then the simultaneous operation of these forces imposes new obligations on physicians and patients as they attempt to arrive at mutually satisfactory decisions. This chapter addressed some of these obligations from the vantage point of theory. I now move from theory to practice in order to explore the relevance of theory to interactions between physicians and patients at the bedside.

VI

Respecting Autonomy: The Obligation for Conversation

PHYSICIANS ARE WELL TRAINED to attend caringly to patients' physical needs. Their education has not prepared them to attend caringly to patients' decision-making needs. Reconciling respect for self-determination with respect for patients' adult and childlike longings is a difficult undertaking. How to achieve such a reconciliation through conversation requires intensive study. In this chapter I shall apply some of the lessons to be learned from the theoretical explorations of the concept of psychological autonomy and the principle of self-determination to clinical situations.

The encounters of Louis Washkansky and Philip Blaiberg—the first and second persons to receive heart transplants—with their surgeon Christiaan Barnard, illustrate the importance of the internal component of self-determination (thinking about choices) for protecting patients' and doctors' psychological autonomy. These clinical examples are dramatic because of the extraordinary nature of the intervention itself, but they are not atypical. The failure to bring significant factors that affect physicians' and patients' choices to self-awareness and to the awareness of the other is common to everyday interactions between physicians and patients. I chose these examples because of the rare availability of reminiscences about the same event by both physician and patient.

The First Two Heart Transplant Patients

I shall begin with Blaiberg's description of his first meeting with Barnard the day after his admission to the hospital:

> . . . I was lying in bed with eyes closed, feeling drowsy and thoroughly miserable when I sensed someone at the head of my bed. I opened my eyes and saw a man. He was tall, young, good-looking with features that reminded me a lot of General Jan Christian Smuts in his later years. His hands were beautiful; the hands of the born surgeon.
> "Don't you know me?" he asked.
> "No, " I said with little interest, "I don't."
> "I'm Professor Chris Barnard," he said.
> "I'm sorry, Professor," I replied, "but I didn't recognize you. I have never seen you in person, and you look so different from your photographs in the Press."
> He spoke earnestly. "Dr. Blaiberg, how do you feel about the prospect of a heart transplant operation? You probably know, don't you, that I am prepared to do you next?"
> "The sooner the better," I said fervently, "and I promise you my full cooperation at all times."
> Though our conversation was brief and he stayed only a few minutes, I was immediately impressed with the stature of the man and his air of buoyant optimism. He inspired me with the greatest confidence, an invaluable asset in the relations between a surgeon and his patient.
> I felt somewhat better. Here was a man to whom I would willingly entrust my life. I came to know him well in the weeks and months that followed. He is a vital, determined, somewhat mercurial, personality, utterly dedicated to his profession.[1]

A few days later, the morning after Washkansky had died, news that had been kept from Blaiberg, Barnard came to see him again. As Blaiberg remembered it,

> [Barnard] was haggard and drawn as though he had not slept all night. He no longer resembled the handsome Smuts, to whom I

had compared him, but more a martyred Christ. I felt a twinge of pity for him when I noticed the pain in his face and eyes. Something, I was sure, had happened to dampen the gaiety and boundless optimism I had seen before

*   *   *

Professor Barnard spoke in low tones. "I feel like a pilot who has just crashed," he said. "Now I want you, Dr. Blaiberg, to help me by taking up another plane as soon as possible to get back my confidence."

Still I did not know what he was driving at. "Professor," I said, puzzled, "why are you telling me this? You know I am prepared to undergo a heart transplant operation at any time you wish."

"But don't you know that Louis Washkansky is dead?" he asked. "He died this morning, of pneumonia."

. . . Now I knew the reason for his distress and agitation.

"Professor Barnard," I said at once, "I want to go through with it now more than ever—not only for my sake but for you and your team who put so much into your effort to save Louis Washkansky."

Blaiberg's description of his initial meeting with Barnard vividly depicts the preemptory emergence of infantile modes of behavior in patients that at least for a while can drown out adult reasoning and reflection. Barnard instantaneously became in Blaiberg's mind an omnipotent parent and hero. He was no longer only a surgeon who would do his level best to prolong life. He also had become a representative of many of the powerful persons Blaiberg had encountered in his life. For example, Barnard became General Smuts, under whom Blaiberg had served and whom he admired greatly. From the first moment he had laid his eyes on Barnard, Blaiberg idealized him. Unquestioning, he placed himself in "the [beautiful] hands of a born surgeon . . . utterly dedicated to his profession," and "willingly [entrusted his] life to him."

In their second meeting, Barnard also became Christ, the powerful protector. Yet, he was the "martyred Christ," who had given His life for the sake of mankind. But it was Blaiberg, not Barnard, who was perhaps prepared to be a martyr for the sake of mankind. Is it not possible that when Blaiberg "noticed the pain in [Barnard's] face and eyes," he unconsciously identified with him, projected his own "distress and agitation" onto Barnard, made him the martyred Christ, and confused his own identity with that of his surgeon? Recall that Blaiberg now wanted to go through with the operation not only for his own sake but for the sake of Barnard and his team as well. If Barnard had suspected that Blaiberg could react in some such fashion, he might have first inquired about how Blaiberg viewed him, and then talked with him about his human limitations as a surgeon, about the limitations of his craft, and, in this instance, about his own uncertainties of providing Blaiberg with the relief that he expected from this novel operation. As a result of such conversations, Blaiberg might eventually have recognized his confusion of Barnard with his life-giving parents, as well as with the real and storybook heroes of his past, and, in turn, placed his surgeon in better perspective.

Patients, particularly those in the throes of serious illness, characteristically become confused about past and present. Barnard's extensive clinical experience must have made him aware of this phenomenon. That he did not attend to it in this instance is another matter. Yet, such inattentiveness raises questions about his responsibilities to recognize such a common reaction, and attempt, through sustained conversations, to moderate Blaiberg's infantile fantasies about him and about the success of the operation. The responsibility for engaging in such conversations cannot be assigned to Blaiberg, it rests with his doctor.

It is most likely, however, that any thoughts Barnard might have entertained of subjecting his patient's magical expectations to reflection and critical appraisal were obliterated by his self-interested eagerness to perform another transplant on a suitable patient as soon as possible. His zeal to forge ahead conflicted with the many doubts Barnard must have entertained about the promise of a procedure never before performed on man. Such disquieting doubts generally tend to be suppressed rather than confronted. They seem to disturb "the courage, grit, or guts" that transplant surgeons have emphasized as being so essential to their work.[2] Yet, as long as such suppressions are deemed essential to effectiveness, they invariably will lead to silence about important matters that deserve discussion.

Thus, another question arises: Was it Barnard's responsibility to become aware of the fact that his own interests might conflict with those of his patient? If he had regarded it as his responsibility, the conflicts would have emerged more readily in conversations with Blaiberg. With some encouragement,

Blaiberg might have raised a number of perplexing and disturbing questions about the operation. Since Barnard did not wish to, or could not, own up to his doubts and conflicts, he surely was not prepared to evoke them in his patient. Instead, he all too quickly said, "[G]ood. I'll come again soon," and took his leave.[3]*

Some time earlier Barnard had similarly avoided conversation with Washkansky's wife, Ann. When she had asked, "What chances do you give him?" he had responded without hesitation or further explanation, "An 80 percent chance." This response was utterly meaningless because neither he nor Ann Washkansky knew what the other meant by "chance." Did it mean Louis' chances of surviving the operation itself, or surviving a few weeks, months, or years after the operation, or of better prospects with or without the operation? Furthermore, "an 80 percent chance" was indefensibly optimistic for any of these categories, given the fact that the operation had never before been performed. Barnard's answer only served the purpose of stopping any self-reflection by doctor or patient and of deflecting any disturbing inquiries by and conversation with Ann Washkansky.

To return to Blaiberg's story, here is Barnard's account of their first meeting:

> I . . . went down to D-I Ward where I found Dr. Blaiberg dozing in bed. He looked like Santa Claus, with a tubby belly, red cheeks, blue ears, and a big mouth—except this was no laughing Santa. His mouth was open and gasping for air.
>
> I nudged him slightly, and he looked at me with elfish eyes.
>
> "Dr. Blaiberg? I've come to introduce myself—or do you know who I am?"
>
> "No, I don't."
>
> "I'm Professor Barnard."
>
> "I'm sorry, Professor . . ."
>
> He gasped for air and continued.
>
> "I should have recognized you . . . I've seen your pictures often . . . but we've never met."
>
> "Well, I've come to say hello and see how you are."
>
> "You can see . . . I'm not well."

In a way, he was worse off than Washkansky had been—especially, in the struggle for air.

"Do you know there's a possibility we can help you by doing a heart transplant on you?"

"Yes, I know."

"How do you feel about that?"

"The sooner, the better . . . I'll co-op . . . cooperate in every way."

I looked into his eyes to see if there was fear. There was none. This was not a fighter like Louis Washkansky. He was not a loner. He was a company man—one of many. But he was without fear, and he believed that we could do it.

"Good," I said. "I'll come again soon."

"Thank you, Professor . . ."

He began to cough and I waited for him to finish.

"The sooner . . . the better," he said.

I returned to my office in the medical school. . . .

Having established by a look into Blaiberg's eyes that there was no fear and by another unidentified process that he was a "company man"—by which Barnard must have meant that Blaiberg had "the interests of the employer rather than those of the workers at heart"[4] and therefore would loyally follow orders —Barnard seemed satisfied. Neither Barnard's nor Blaiberg's reminiscences mention any further conversations between them about the impending heart transplantation.

Barnard's initial conversation with Louis Washkansky, although somewhat more extensive than the one with Blaiberg, was equally devoid of any exploration of their respective expectations, fears, and hopes. Dr. Kaplan, Washkansky's family physician, had urged Barnard to explain the heart transplant operation to Washkansky and this was one of the ostensible reasons for his first visit. According to Barnard, he found Washkansky "propped up in bed, reading a book":

"Mr. Washkansky, I have come to introduce myself. I believe Dr. Kaplan and Professor Schrire have spoken to you about it—we intend doing a heart transplant on you, and for this you will be admitted to my ward."

"That's fine with me—I'm ready and waiting for it."

"If you like, I can tell you what we know and what we don't know about this."

He nodded and waited for me to go on. He was obviously very

sick, but you could see he had once been quite strong and good-looking. There were also the features of a generous man—a large mouth with the face folds of one who smiled often. He had big ears and big hands, and his eyes, peering at me over the spectacles, were gray-green—and waiting. So, I spoke to him.

"We know you have a heart disease for which we can do nothing more. You have had all possible treatment, and you are getting no better. We can put a normal heart into you, after taking out your heart that's no longer any good, and there's a chance you can get back to normal life again."

"So they told me. So I'm ready to go ahead."

He said no more. His eyes remained on me but with no indication he wanted to know any more.

"Well, then . . . good-bye," I said.

"Good-bye."

As I turned to go, he began reading again. It was a Western. How, I wondered, could he return to pulp fiction after being suddenly cast into the greatest drama of his life? What was it about human nature that caused such a reaction? No man in the history of the world had ever met the surgeon who was going to cut out his heart and replace it with a new human one—at least, not until this moment, which was now being lost somewhere in a Western novel.

What had made him turn away? He was a realist. He carried no false illusions, no special clouds of rationale. He lived for the moment, for the hour, for the full living of all of it. And now, I had offered him just that—life. Yet he had not asked the odds, nor any details.[5]

Washkansky's apparent disinterest in learning more about the operation disturbed Barnard momentarily. However, he brushed aside his concerns over Washkansky's puzzling behavior and concluded instead that "nothing more, no words were needed."

Should Barnard have insisted that more was needed, that they had to talk with one another so that both would know, for example, that he was offering Washkansky only the possibility, but surely no promise, of life? Should he have insisted that they talk more, particularly in this instance, since "[N]o man in the history of the world had ever met the surgeon who was going to cut out his heart"? Should he have inquired why Washkansky who would soon come face to face with the "greatest drama of his life" returned "to pulp fiction"?

In raising these issues, I do not question that ultimately

Washkansky might have made the same choice. I only question the nature and quality of Barnard's and Washkansky's thinking about available choices. Both, at best, had reflected on the forthcoming operation in isolation, and neither had any idea what had transpired in the other's mind. At the least, respect for Washkansky's psychological autonomy required Barnard to challenge his patient's silent acquiescence. In this case, where the patient was especially needy and was surrounded by seemingly powerful healers, his hopes, fears and magical expectations should not have been left unexplored.

If Washkansky wanted a new heart, he also had to have the heart to learn more about the operation. The first heart transplant was an extraordinary procedure. In selecting an appropriate patient, Barnard needed to pay attention not only to Washkansky's physical suitability for undergoing the operation but also to Washkansky's capacity to understand the consequences. Any patient who did not meet the latter criterion was not a suitable candidate for the first transplanted heart. In more ordinary situations, as I have suggested in the previous chapter, a patient's waiver of disclosure and consent may be more acceptable after a prior inquiry into his reasons. Washkansky's operation, however, was not an ordinary event. The inattentiveness to conversation in this instance, which made meaningful consent impossible, only underscores its general disregard in physician-patient interactions.

The silence about airing important concerns on the part of both parties is strikingly illustrated in Barnard's second meeting with Blaiberg. Washkansky had died in the meantime and Barnard asked for Blaiberg's help in "taking up another plane . . . to get back my confidence." Barnard apparently did not ask himself first whether his patently self-interested request—particularly the way he expressed it—was an appropriate one. Should he have known that unless he carefully distinguished between his interests and those of his patient, neither he nor Blaiberg could ever be sure whether consent to the surgery was given more for Blaiberg's own sake or for that of Barnard and his team? One example of such confusion is Blaiberg's statement that he wanted to go through with the operation because Barnard had already put so much "effort [into saving] Louis Washkansky."

While the rational and irrational expectations and their impact on the interactions between Barnard, Washkansky and

Blaiberg clearly emerge in their personal reminiscences of their meetings, these expectations were never identified; they were passed over in silence. The process of thinking about choices was given all too short shrift. Thus another question arises: To what extent must physicians as well as patients subject their motivations and expectations to reflection and critical appraisal prior to and during their encounters?

Barnard's reminiscences give no indication that he engaged in self-reflection in order to sort out his conflicts of interest. He did admit to being severely shaken by Washkansky's death and to guilt. He told both Blaiberg and his friend and fellow-surgeon Jacques Roux, "I crash-landed." Indeed, Barnard entertained the idea of not performing another heart transplant. He did not consider sharing his doubts with Blaiberg, however, when he finally decided to proceed and went to Blaiberg to ask for his help.

Immediately after Washkansky's death, Barnard briefly withdrew into himself. Roux's comforting words that he "had opened the way for others" did not console him. Instead, he accused himself:

> No, Jacques, we crashed because of my mistakes. I should not have used cobalt treatment. I gave too many antirejection drugs. He got an infection because we lowered his resistance too much. And we didn't correctly diagnose that, until too late. . . . Even with what we know now, it'll still be working in the dark and I've lost my nerve. I'm afraid, Jacques. I'm afraid of the dark.

At the subsequent autopsy, still depressed over his failure, Barnard's spirits lifted quickly once the pathologist pointed to the implanted heart:

> "Chris," he said. "These suture lines are perfect—there's not an error or a clot anywhere. It's beautiful."
>
> I looked from him to the other faces around the table. Each one nodded, or in some way said to me: "Well done, Chris."
>
> At that moment I had my answer and I began to build again. I had not failed. I had succeeded. The first attempt, with all its pain and sorrow, had been made for the second. To now turn back would be to deny the first—*to turn away from Louis Washkansky's dream.*
>
> Leaving the postmortem with Jacques, I said I was going to do another transplant.

"What's more," I said. "I'm going to America and appear on 'Face the Nation.' I'm going to face the world—and then come back and do a transplant on Dr. Blaiberg."

"Provided Dr. Blaiberg is still willing," said Jacques.

"Yes," I said. "And I'd better *find that out* right now."

When I reached the ward Dr. Blaiberg was awake, and his wife, Eileen, was sitting with him. . . .

* * * *

"Dr. Blaiberg, do you know that Mr. Washkansky died this morning?"

"No, I didn't know it."

"I didn't tell him," said his wife. "I didn't know how to tell him."

"I expected it," he said. "I've been listening to the radio . . . I knew how ill he was."

"I've come to tell you why he died and what we found on examining him."

Dr. Blaiberg nodded and his wife held his hand.

"He died of pneumonia, and there was no evidence, as far as we could see, of a failure of the transplanted heart. But the transplant was a failure anyway, because we kept him alive for only eighteen days. So if you don't want to have your operation, you don't have to go through with it. It's for you to decide."

"Professor . . ."

He stopped to glance at his wife, then continued.

"I want to be a well man, and if I'm not well, I'd rather be dead. How soon can you do the next transplant?"

"Thank you."

"How soon can you do it?"

"I have to go overseas for about ten days, but we'll do it as soon as possible after I come back. In the meantime, I'll have you transferred to my ward."

"More than ever," he said, "I want this to be a success—not only for my sake, but also for you and the other doctors."

"You can help us by doing one thing."

"Yes—what is it?"

"Stay alive until I get back."

"Don't worry," he said. "You'll find me here—waiting."

Barnard's depiction of his goal as fulfilling ''Washkansky's dream'' is startling and suggests that he was as confused about his identity as Blaiberg was about his own. The dream that now propelled Barnard to go on was no longer his, but Washkansky's!

Barnard's difficulty in distinguishing himself from Washkansky probably was influenced by guilt and sadness over Washkansky's death and by a wish to bring him back to life intrapsychically by making a common cause with "Washkansky's dream." At the same time he also must have been angry at Washkansky for having abandoned him—a common grief reaction among mourners who have lost an important person. He displaced his anger onto Blaiberg by abandoning him for ten days in order to "Face the Nation." Even though Barnard's trip to New York was motivated by other reasons as well, it may not be too far fetched to speculate that his anger at Washkansky for dying played a role in his leaving Blaiberg at this crucial moment.

Let me offer another speculation: Barnard may also have needed proof that Blaiberg would turn out to be a better patient than Washkansky, by "[staying] alive until [he got] back." If Blaiberg could accomplish that feat then perhaps he would stay around longer after the operation than Washkansky had. If this speculation has merit, it only proves that physicians are not exempt from magical thinking.

The needs and wishes of Barnard, Blaiberg and even a dead Washkansky became hopelessly intertwined in Barnard's mind. In Barnard's and his patients' dreams about the operation, an identity of interest could readily be taken for granted. If their dreams had been subjected to the harsh reality of waking thought, however, their conflicting interests would have become apparent. Guided too much by dreams, Barnard remained unaware of the potential conflicts between his own interests and those of his patients. Had he paused and reflected, he might have been able to separate his interests from theirs as they affected his thinking about the available choices as well as about the ultimate decision. Since he did not, he could neither explore them with himself nor consider informing Blaiberg about his doubts about the operation that he had shared earlier with his friend Roux.

Like so many physicians, Barnard assumed that his interests were the same as those of his patients and thus felt no hesitation to acting on behalf of Washkansky and Blaiberg. Respect for their psychological autonomy, however, would have demanded that Barnard keep his and their identities separate in order to explore their individual hopes and fears about the operation. Some might contend that the patients' necessitous and precarious conditions made any committed effort by Barnard to explain himself and his operation futile and irrelevant. The patients' self-inflicted coercions and magical expectations, however, must also be evaluated in terms of Barnard's contribution to the final outcome. His silence about crucial matters and his own magical expectations about the operation powerfully affected his patients' choices. Recall, for example, that Barnard told Blaiberg and his wife that "Washkansky had died of *pneumonia* and [that] there was no evidence, as far as we could see, of a failure of the transplanted heart." Yet to his friend Roux he had spoken of "still working in the dark," of having given "too many antirejection drugs," and of having "lowered [Washkansky's] resistance too much."

Necessitous conditions notwithstanding, Barnard should at least have made an effort to inform his patients about what he knew and did not know about heart transplant operations and then to identify and clarify any misconceptions and distortions in their responses to his invitation of joining him in this great adventure. Even if his patients had initially resisted his invitation to converse and think together, Barnard should have insisted that they talk for a while. The inevitable conflict that such insistence creates between the values of autonomy and privacy should be resolved in favor of autonomy. Such invasions of privacy must be tolerated in order to enhance patients' psychological autonomy through insight and not allow it to be further undermined by too hopeful promises, blind misconceptions, and false certainties.

John Stuart Mill's words bear repeating: "Considerations to aid his judgment, exhortations to strengthen his will, may be offered to him, even obtruded on him, by others: but he himself is the final judge."[6] Mill appreciated the need for conversation. Respect for psychological autonomy finds expression in the first part of Mill's recommendation, in being attentive to the vulnerabilities of the process of thinking about choices. Respect for individual rights finds expression in Mill's second assertion that patients' ultimate choices must be honored. These distinctions, introduced in Chapter V, may clarify the common clinical controversy over whether physicians should respect either patients' "*rights*" or "*needs*." Insisting on conversation and reflection expresses a concern for patients' needs. The ultimate acceptance of their choices expresses a respect for their rights.

Transference and Countertransference in Physician-Patient Interactions

Respectful conversation between physicians and patients requires an appreciation of one particular set of irrational feelings that both bring to their encounters with one another. These irrationalities manifest themselves most dramatically, on the part of patients, in an over-evaluation of the physician as an omnipotent healer and, on the part of physicians, in an under-evaluation of the patient as a competent adult. The recurrent emergence of such feelings in all physician-patient interactions bears testimony to the existence of psychological vulnerabilities inherent in human beings that only become magnified in the presence of uncertainty over health and cure. As the encounters between Barnard and his patients demonstrate, these irrational forces need to be better understood and better managed if disclosure and consent are to have any meaning. A comment by Leonardo da Vinci about the distinctions between painting and sculpting is apposite here. He wrote that in sculpting—*per via di levare*—the figures come into being by chiselling away "the distortions" introduced by the material; on the other hand, in painting—*per via di porre*—the painter adds his own "distortions" to the canvas.[7] In conversing with patients, doctors must take great care to eliminate as far as possible the patient's distortions without adding their own to them. I shall explore patients' distortions first.

Transference

Early in his work with patients, Freud observed the development of an "intense emotional relationship between the patient and the analyst which [cannot] be accounted for by the actual situation."[8] He noted that "[i]t can be of a positive or of a negative character and can vary between the extreme of a passionate, completely sensual love and the unbridled expression of an embittered defiance and hatred." He called this phenomenon, of which patients initially are largely unaware, "transference." By this term he sought to capture patients' proclivity to endow their analyst with many of the characteristics of their earliest caretakers rather than to view the analyst solely as who he is. The process of transference leads patients to project onto the analyst all kinds of magical expectations, hopes, and fears that are intrinsically irrational because they emerge out of confusion not only of past and present but also of fantasy and reality.[9]

Freud appreciated that transference was not limited to psychoanalytic treatment. The special sensory deprivations that patients are asked to tolerate in psychoanalysis—for example, not being able to see the analyst while lying on the couch—only make transference manifestations more conspicuous. He noted that "it is a universal phenomenon of the human mind, it decides the success of all medical influence, and in fact dominates the whole of each person's relations to his human environment."[10] Since human beings bring to all their interactions residues of earlier experiences, transference is a quite normal phenomenon that affects every human relationship.

Transference feelings become more intense when persons are ill and beset by fears and anxieties. Patients' basic modes of expression of such feelings are in many ways predictable and stereotypical, but their finely tuned manifestations also reveal facets of an individual's uniqueness and essence, of his or her personality as it has evolved in interactions with parents and other important persons during childhood years. Thus, manifestations of transference constitute a mixture of highly individualized personal reactions, as well as universal human adult and childlike longings, that possess both rational and irrational components. Transferences can guide and misguide persons—the latter more in times of stress, when infantile hopes and fears surface most insistently.

In clinical settings, even when there have been prior disappointments with other doctors, patients' transferences tend to be positive at first. Patients' hopes that they have finally found an all-comforting parent-caretaker who will relieve all suffering, spring eternal. And so do doctors' hopes that they have finally met a trusting and uncomplaining child-patient. In the face of such heady expectations on both sides, their initial meetings generally turn out to be quite congenial and satisfying. Patients' enormous expectations of having met at last a totally dedicated doctor who will cure all their ills, however, can rarely, if ever, be fulfilled. When disappointments set in, they become magnified by patients' negative transference feelings. These, too, are universal, although during the initial encounters between doctor and patient such negative feelings may be overshadowed by positive ones.

Early manifestations of negative transference may go unnoticed. These negative feelings also are rooted in early memories—found even among those raised under the most ideal circumstances—of frustration and discomfort, which evoked in the infant a momentary but overwhelming sense of despair. Parents cannot always sense all their infants' needs and infants are most vulnerable to feelings of despair over relatively innocuous and short-lived deprivations. Thus, individuals' earliest experiences create two contradictory convictions: that caretakers will protect them as once upon a time their all-powerful parents did, and that such hopes are doomed to inevitable disappointment. Deep feelings of basic trust and mistrust are the legacy of all human beings. Magical and hopeful expectations exist side by side with expectations of cruel disappointment.

Once the universal presence of such contradictory and conflicted, magical and realistic, hopeful and hopeless expectations is recognized, it should come as no surprise that these fulfilled and unfulfilled feelings left over from earlier years are unloaded onto physicians. These feelings manifest themselves often only subtly and surreptiously, in conduct that contains confusing admixtures of childlike surrender and childlike rebelliousness. A better appreciation of these proclivities by physicians might prevent their being seduced by their patients' apparent initial willingness to submit unconditionally to their parent-doctors. Instead, doctors might take greater care preparing for the moment of inevitable disappointment by challenging patients' readiness to put themselves in their doctors' hands without question. If doctors were to recognize that patients' magical expectations must be moderated by confronting patients with medical realities, then physicians might more carefully combine expressions of hope with a more realistic appraisal of patients' conditions.

Physicians need to appreciate that they are not only the victims of these transferences but also their abettors. Because they have been as blind to the existence of transference as their patients, doctors have encouraged and augmented patients' transference feelings by unwittingly promising more than they can deliver or by not confronting their patients' explicit and implicit unrealistic expectations. A greater awareness by both parties of the power of transference and the obligation to contain its power are essential preconditions for conversation. Initially, this obligation must be assumed by professionals rather than by their patients. Patients can only learn of the power of transference over time and through personal experiences with aware physicians who educate them about its manifestations.

Transference manifestations, however, cannot be eliminated; they can only be attenuated. For example, physicians generally make their treatment recommendation immediately after completing the diagnostic work-up and without a prior exploration of patients' views on the need for and choice of treatment. Under the influence of transference, patients often respond to recommendations with a premature acceptance or rejection of the proposed intervention that later may come to haunt the physician-patient relationship. Particularly in the case of acceptance, agreement and surrender may imperceptibly blend in patients' minds, and subsequently become affected by doubts and even convictions that it was solely the doctor's judgment that led to the treatment. Therefore unawareness of the transference may lead patients to believe that an intervention was coerced by their doctors even when physicians had no intention to force compliance. Yet, in a real sense, the agreement was also coerced by doctors' inattentiveness to the influence of transference reactions on patients' agreement to the proposed treatment. Patients' subsequent hostile reactions are evidence not only of patients' ''ungratefulness,'' but also of their iatrogenic responses to a justified feeling of having been seduced into following doctors' (parents') orders in the first place. That patients were, in a sense, also the authors of the coercion matters little because, as I have already noted, the management of transference is first of all the responsibility of physicians.

Transference reactions can be reduced to more manageable proportions when one is aware of their existence. Awareness itself could lessen physicians' temptation to contribute to the regressive pull either actively, by treating patients as children, or passively, by keeping patients in the dark and not inviting their participation in decision making. Indeed, patients' transference reactions have reinforced physicians' traditional view of patients' incompetence. Under the domination of transference, patients do appear more childlike than they actually are or necessarily need to be. Physicians have been blinded by these ubiquitous and spontaneous manifestations of transference and have not seen that patients are not children. If doctors were more aware of transference, they would more readily discern that underneath the manifestations of childlike behavior there exists a mature adult patient. Doctors would then be more inclined to learn how to address and nurture the intact, mature parts of patients' functioning and how to reverse the regressive pull engendered by illness and its attendant anxieties. Anna Freud tried to teach these lessons of transference to students at Case Western Reserve Medical School by reminding them that

> . . . [t]he patient . . . will do his best to push you into the place of parental authority, and he will make use of you as a parental authority to the utmost. You must understand that. On the other hand, you must not be tempted to treat him as a child. You must be tolerant towards him as you would be towards a child and as respectful as you would be towards a fellow adult because he has only gone back to childhood as far as he's ill. He also has another part of his personality which has remained intact, and that part of him will resent it deeply, if you make too much use of your authority. . . .[11]

Misled by the phenomenon of transference, physicians have thought that patients wanted them to assume complete authority. Therefore physicians issued orders. When such orders turned patients even more into children—submissive or obstreperous ones—doctors did not separate the contributions that the disease, the physician, and the patient made to the regression. Traditional patterns of interactions between physicians and their patients have made childlikeness a self-fulfilling prophecy.

The phenomenon of transference reinforces the need for formulating a concept of autonomy that takes human psychology into account. Patients' confusion between past and present, present and past, parental figures and doctors, and doctors and parental figures affects autonomous functioning in significant ways. Respect for patients' autonomy and self-determination requires that physicians become more real to their patients. Doctors must learn to distinguish themselves with greater deliberateness from parental imagoes who, in time distant, often had to issue commands rather than explanations. To so distinguish themselves, doctors must learn to acknowledge their limitations and the limitations of medicine, to be sensitive to any emergence of magical expectations in their patients, and to try to correct such expectations by explaining what an intervention can and cannot accomplish. In short, doctors must address the irrational and unconscious expectations of patients that inform the choice-making process. Such efforts will not always meet with success and, indeed, can never be totally successful. However hard one tries to be true to Rousseau's aphorism that "It is better to know one's chains than to deck them with flowers,"[12] some chains that imprison the human mind inevitably remain decked with flowers.

To make the process of thinking about choices less coercive, however, physicians must respect patients' ultimate choices even if they believe that such choices will have unfortunate consequences for their patients. At times, doctors may have to agree to do less than they would like to do; at other times they regretfully may have to terminate the relationship. These are difficult decisions, but if thinking about choices is seen as an opportunity to exert an influence on patients, it must be done in the spirit of ultimately respecting patients' choices. Otherwise thinking together about choices becomes at best meaningless and at worst a cruel hoax.

Countertransference

Irrational and unconscious expectations influence physicians' conduct as well. Early in his explorations, Freud recognized that doctors' unconscious has an impact on their relations with patients, and he gave these manifestations the name "countertransference."[13] Psychoanalysts, however, have not paid the same attention to this phenomenon as they have to transference. There is a striking paucity of literature on countertransference as compared to the vast literature on transference. Moreover, reading the few articles on countertransference reveals the remarkable fact that psychoanalysts have largely attributed the emergence of troublesome countertransference reactions to patients. Countertransference has been defined in the psychoanalytic literature as reactions in the therapist engendered *by* the patient. Although psychoanalysts have paid more attention to countertransference than have other physicians, psychoanalysts have fallen into the trap of generally imputing the source of irrationality engendered in the therapeutic settings to patients. It is the patient who is identified as the prime mover of what is unleashed in the therapist. Always the patient!

Countertransference accompanies physicians as much on their daily rounds as transference accompanies patients to hospitals and doctors' offices. Indeed, the longer I reflect upon the idea of informed consent, the more convinced I become that professionals' unrecognized countertransferences are a greater impediment to its meaningful implementation than are patients' transferences. Roy Menninger stated this well:

> . . . [T]he doctor has too much narcissistic investment in his power position vis-a-vis the patient. Many of us have developed subtle but disguised ways of maintaining that power position, all in the name of "good treatment." The fact is that medicine, as many of us practice it, encourages a patient's dependency. It does not encourage a more desirable goal, namely the establishment of a kind of parity in the relationship that promotes a greater responsibility by the patient for his own treatment. . . . Physicians generally do not give enough attention to the need for enabling, encouraging, promoting patients to establish a greater sense of individual control, a sense of mastery, through a kind of therapeutic alliance rather than a therapeutic autocracy that is psychologically and economically gratifying to the physician. I am well aware that our patients are expert at putting us in a position narcissistically satisfying to us, making it thereby more difficult to recognize this problem and to change it. . . .[14]

On the other hand, consider the implications of Brian Bird's diametrically different view on professional authority which is more in tune with prevailing professional attitudes. In his book, *Talking with Patients*, he wrote:

> . . . Talking with patients, like the whole business of being a doctor, is a very large order. Just how big, and just what it all consists of, no one really knows.
>
> One little understood thing that distinguishes being a doctor from not being one is the position a doctor assumes relative to people who come to him for help. The doctor's way of responding to requests for help is his special thing; it is a quality that transcends knowledge, a quality that demands a unique sense of responsibility for human life, a responsibility built on an almost arrogant kind of confidence in himself, a quality that has evolved from the age-old tradition of patient care.
>
> [H]e must accept within himself the seemingly arrogant idea

that he has the power, the right, the authority to do the unusual, peculiar things "being a doctor" demands of him. . . . This final authority must come from him; he must have the nerve, the confidence, the gall, or whatever it takes, to grant it unto himself.

. . . Ordinary people do ordinary things. Only extraordinary people do extraordinary things. It is in this sense that doctors are indeed special. They are special, not because they are more intelligent, more capable, more trustworthy, or more anything else, but because the public has given them this extraordinary role and they have accepted it. . . .[15]

The implications of Bird's view make the title of his book misleading. Talking *with* patients is impossible if the sweeping and unqualified prerogatives Bird has delegated to physicians continue to rule the interactions between them and their patients.

Moreover, it is not at all clear whether "the power, the right, [and] the authority" have been given to doctors by the public or whether "this extraordinary role" was imposed on and passively accepted by the public. Whatever its origins, the professional conduct depicted by Bird is deeply ingrained in the ethos of physicians. Since such conduct has generally been considered appropriate professional behavior, its rationality has not been questioned. Yet could not such professional conduct be as irrational as doctors' personal conduct at times turns out to be?

Take Bird's view of arrogance as an example. Some psychoanalysts would consider personal arrogance as a countertransference reaction, but they might not so view it if arrogance were deemed to be an essential professional attribute. Yet, are arrogance and many other so-called essential professional attributes indispensable characteristics of professionals or are they acquired characteristics that serve physicians' personal needs more than their professional ones? While personal and professional needs are interrelated, they deserve separate consideration so that one can identify in particular the irrational components of professional conduct. Irrationality in physicians' conduct can easily become obscured by deeming it essential to the proper exercise of one's professional responsibilities.

A broader definition of countertransference that encompasses not only physicians' personal conduct but also their deeply ingrained professional attitudes toward patients will move to center stage a re-examination of the impact on physician-patient interactions of a great many unquestioned professional attitudes.

These attitudes include the need to appear authoritative, the importance of hiding uncertainties from patients, the need to view patients as incompetent to participate in decision making, and the belief that patients' welfare depends on patients' trusting doctors' capacities to know what is in patients' best interests. A re-examination of such basic professional convictions will not be easy, for professionals are unaccustomed to looking that deeply into their professional psyche. As Freud suggested, it is difficult enough for professionals to take a look at personal neurotic blindspots. At a minimum, however, it must be recognized that many of the attributes of a good physician enumerated by Bird must be drastically modified if disclosure and consent are ever to become meaningful obligations. An ''arrogant kind of confidence'' does not invite mutual decision making.

My broader view of countertransference suggests that not only physicians' personal beliefs but also their professional beliefs are influenced by irrational and unconscious factors. Indeed, the most pernicious countertransference problem may turn out to be that in their professional interactions with patients, physicians view themselves as too rational and their patients as too irrational. A more realistic view of the balance between rationality and irrationality in both parties will itself improve decision making between physicians and patients. The projection of irrationalities originating within physicians onto patients may prove to be one of the most pervasive and fateful countertransference reactions.

Professional Education for Decision Making

A greater awareness of the complex interrelationship between rationality and irrationality in professional conduct could lead to curricular reforms that will offer medical students the opportunity to explore the impact of personal and professional beliefs on their interactions with patients. I do not advocate probing and exploring students' personal motivations, as this is an individual and private matter, but rather, exploring the important though neglected topic of professional responsibility. Different views about the nature of medical practice, about doctors' perceived mission, and attitudes toward patients decisively shape professional behavior and deserve scrutiny.

For example, students can be alerted to the fact that doctors are not exempt from resorting to disguised magical thinking when, as so frequently happens in the fight against disease, their scientific medical knowledge and skills prove impotent against the claims of nature. At such times, all kinds of senseless interventions are tried in an unconscious effort to cure the incurable magically through a "wonder drug," a novel surgical procedure, or a penetrating psychological interpretation. At least medical students can learn to appreciate that it may be their magical hopes that cause them to intervene, rather than believing that they are responding to the magical expectations of their patients. Thus doctors' heroic attempts to try anything may not necessarily be responsive to patients' needs but may turn out to be a projection of their own needs onto patients. Students might then also learn how to ascertain through conversation with their patients whether it is their or their patients' expectations that propel them to act.

At first glance, it seems surprising that doctors are so inattentive to their personal and professional blindspots, idiosyncracies, and biases. One must remember, however, that recognition of the impact of professional irrationalities on physician-patient relations would expose doctors' vulnerabilities to irrational and unconscious thinking in the decision-making process, in what they disclose and do not disclose to patients. Physicians dread recognizing these irrationalities; since they are unaccustomed to and uncomfortable with probing their conduct, they prefer to attribute irrational conduct primarily to patients.

A better appreciation of physicians' and patients' mutual vulnerabilities would decisively affect conversations between them. This is not to suggest that they engage in a psychoanalytic exploration of their motivations and expectations. A psychoanalytic understanding of how past and present have shaped patients' individual personalities is not possible in non-psychotherapeutic settings. What is an attainable goal, however, is a greater awareness that these competing forces do in fact exist and that they shape all conduct in known *and* unknown ways. An equally attainable goal is for patients and physicians to assume the mutual obligation of engaging in conversation, to *con-scire* (to know together)—the root verb of the word "conscious" and "conscience"—about what they want of and can do for one another.[16]

To think and to converse with patients meaningfully and effectively, physicians must be more self-reflective and sort out competing personal and professional values that may affect their recommendations before they make them. The story of Iphigenia in Chapter IV is an example of the impact of a surgeon's ill-sorted out personal and professional judgments and self-interests on his disclosures to and interactions with a patient. Physicians also must assist patients to distinguish unrealistic and too hopeful expectations from more realistic ones. Both parties must make an effort to expose to scrutiny their doubts, fears, distortions, misconceptions, uncertainties and plain ignorance. Since they can never be fully exposed or clarified, however, nagging questions will always remain about the influence of unconscious, irrational and just plain unconsidered thoughts and feelings on physician-patient deliberations and final decisions. These nagging questions can serve as an important corrective for both parties, for it will make them appreciate that certainty is hard to come by, that in case of disagreement neither physician nor patient can be sure about who is correct. If then there is still time, both parties may seize the opportunity to reflect further about their different views on the matter before them.

What I propose is a difficult and ambitious assignment, but not an impossible one. Education can go a long way toward improving current deficiencies in physician-patient conversation. While medical training for technical competence has improved enormously during this century, training for decision-making competence has not been given nearly the same attention. Proper professional training must encompass this dimension. How to converse must be taught just as thoroughly as principles of surgery and medicine, for by now I hope that I have scuttled the prevailing notion that what constitutes proper professional conduct with respect to decision making is so self-evident that it does not require formal instruction. The complexities of decision making and choice defy such an assertion.

One must also question a related argument against such training: that the establishment of general principles for decision making is irrelevant for medical practice because every patient is unique and presents a unique problem. This argument makes too much of individual differences. What is true for the treatment of physical diseases is equally applicable for decision making. With respect to the former, principles of customary practice have always alerted doctors that any contemplated deviation from such principles must first be carefully evaluated and justified; the intent behind this admonition is to safeguard patients against reckless experimentation and treatment.

Similarly, my prior discussion of transference and countertransference intended to demonstrate that, individual differences notwithstanding, all patients and physicians react in common and predictable ways whenever they communicate with one another. We need to formulate principles based on an understanding of the psychology of physicians and patients and on notions about proper professional conduct with respect to decision making. Guided by such principles, physicians will be alerted to pause and reflect on the reasons for any deviation from them in individual situations. For example, let us assume that it becomes proper practice for physicians not only to present to patients their choice of treatment but also to explain carefully alternative treatments. Then, whenever physicians give short shrift to alternatives, they will be alerted that they may not be guided by sound professional reasons (although it may turn out that they are), but rather, by personal considerations or special concerns about this particular patient that require separate evaluation. Or, let us assume that it becomes proper practice for physicians to be wary of a too ready acquiescence by patients to their recommendations, particularly when the proposed intervention involves considerable risks. Then, whenever patients too readily agree, doctors may be more inclined to explore with patients the possible influence on the latter's conduct of misconceptions or magical expectations about the proposed procedure.

Doctors and patients are subject to the influence of irrational motivations that are difficult to identify in individual situations and therefore readily subject to rationalizations. The establishment of general principles for the conduct of conversations between physicians and patients in average expectable situations will provide important cautionary signals whenever one or the other departs or wishes to depart from customary conduct. Such contemplated deviations will alert physicians to the need either for additional reflection about the possible impact of idiosyncratic personal and professional considerations on their recommendations or for additional probing of patients' expectations. Conversations under the aegis of principles do not undermine respect for patients' individuality. The opposite is true. Guided by principles, patients' individuality can be better recognized and protected from physicians' unexamined value judgments.

Choice and Responsibility

I now turn to the decision itself, to choice, the external component of self-determination. Patients' ultimate choices deserve the utmost respect, even given the fact that illness can impair their optimal psychological functioning. Unless patients' regressive manifestations are moderated through conversation, they should not serve as justification for imposing doctors' authority on the final decision, if only because coercion in the name of psychological health can easily run wild. Thus in the evaluation of patients' ultimate choices, considerations of human beings' psychological limitations should not lead to overruling patients' decisions. Although this may mean bowing at times to "foolish" choices, they must be honored to protect the process of thinking about choices which would become compromised if the threat of having patients' choices vetoed whenever they appear foolish hangs over their heads.

If the process of thinking about choices is attended to with care, the problem of a total stand-off between physicians and patients may turn out to be a rare event. In making this prediction I do not wish to suggest that patients will always follow doctors' recommendations or that doctors will or should honor all patients' requests, but rather, that in the face of disagreement both may discover through conversation that their "irreconcilable" differences have merit if viewed from the other's perspective and that both views deserve respect.

The process of thinking about choices can only be effectively carried out if physicians and patients are expected to take responsibility for their conduct and if both affirm that they must be allowed to carry out this responsibility in their own ways and must accept responsibility for their own mistakes. The idea that human beings are responsible for their choices comports with my views on psychological autonomy. Its underlying assumption that human thought and action are shaped by rational and irrational, conscious and unconscious motivations and expectations, only invites postulating an obligation for human beings to learn how to own up better to their unconscious, their irrationalities, their passions, and their impulses. Human beings' impulses are *their* impulses, their unconscious is *their* unconscious and they need not necessarily be defeated by their impulses' imperious demands. Indeed if persons were to acknowledge their impulses and their unconscious as their own, their chances of controlling them would often be greatly improved. As Loewald has put it, "to so acknowledge, recognize and understand one's unconscious . . . means to move from a position of passivity in relation to it to a position where active care of it becomes possible, where it becomes a task worthy of pursuit to make one's own business and concern those needs and wishes, fantasies, conflicts and traumatic events and defenses which have been passively experienced and reproduced."[17]

Freud once observed that the importance psychoanalysis attributes to the influence of the unconscious on thought and action dealt a grave blow to human beings' self-esteem by asserting that persons are not complete masters of their own "ego." Freud's observation can be extended in another direction. However great a mortification of human narcissism, the greater burden which acceptance of the unconscious imposes on human beings may be the concomitant responsibility of attending to the impact of unconscious impulses on conduct. If that responsibility were accepted, human beings would have to pause and reflect prior to action. Old verities that an appreciation of the conscious determinants of behavior is the hallmark of responsibility would become suspect. Instead, human beings would have to appreciate that they are condemned (or liberated) to live life with a perpetual sense of healthy scepticism about their capacities to know fully why, in particular situations, they wish to act one way rather than another. Such insights would give additional support to the recommendations I have made for thinking about choices. Doctors and patients would appreciate that conversation serves the function of increasing both parties' responsibility for their conduct, not by analyzing irrationalities in any depth, but by clarifying misconceptions and misunderstandings. To do that much requires an awareness that rationality and irrationality, transference and countertransference affect psychological autonomy and, in turn, choice.

Overruling Patients' Choices

Despite all that I have said so far, *rare* situations may arise when patients' choices should not be honored. The encounter between Mark Siegler and his patient, Mr. D., may be an example in point. Some years ago, while an attending physician at a teaching hospital, Siegler met Mr. D., a previously healthy 66-year-old black man who had come to the emergency room suffering from an acute febrile illness of three day's duration.[18] He seemed critically ill and was admitted to one of the medical wards. A chest X-ray demonstrated a generalized pneumonia and he was treated aggressively with three antibiotics. The next day his condition worsened and his physicians concluded that two uncomfortable but relatively routine diagnostic procedures—a bronchial brushing to obtain a small sample of lung tissue and a bone marrow examination—might establish the cause of his illness. The patient refused permission for performing these tests and, when his physicians repeatedly attempted to explain their necessity, Mr. D. "became angry and agitated by this prolonged pressure and subsequently began refusing even routine blood tests and X-rays."

A psychiatric consultant found him competent and concluded "that Mr. D. understood the severity of his illness . . . and that he was making a rational choice in refusing the tests." The patient's condition deteriorated and 24 hours later he appeared to be near death. He then refused to be placed on a respirator and during two forty-five minute interviews at the bedside, Siegler was unable to get Mr. D. to change his mind. At the same time everything that Mr. D. had said convinced Siegler

> that he understood the gravity of his situation. For example, when I told him he was dying, he replied: "Everyone has to die. If I die now, I am ready." When I asked him if he came to the hospital to be helped, he stated: "I want to be helped. I want you to treat me with whatever medicine you think I need. I don't want any more tests and I don't want the breathing machine."
>
> I gradually became convinced that despite the severity of his illness and his high fever, he was making a conscious, rational decision to selectively refuse a particular kind of treatment. In view of the frankness of our discussion, I then asked him whether he would want us to resuscitate him if he had a cardiorespiratory arrest. He

turned away and said: "We've been through this before; now leave me alone." I left the bedside.

*   *   *   *

Mr. D. soon became semi-conscious and had a cardiorespiratory arrest. Despite the objections of the houseofficers, I did not attempt to resuscitate him, and he died.

Siegler identified six factors that influenced his decision "to support [Mr. D.'s] choices": (1) "the patient's ability to make (rational) choices about his care," based on an assessment of whether a patient has "retained sufficient intellect and rationality to make choices"; (2) "the nature of the person making the choice," based on the doctor's knowledge about the patient's "personality, character, ideas and beliefs"—in short on an assessment of whether the patient is "acting autonomously—that is, with authenticity and independence"; (3) "the attitudes and values of the physician responsible for the decision"; (4) "the patient's age"; (5) "the nature of the illness" (its prognosis and treatability); and (6) "the clinical setting in which the physician works."

Siegler's decision to defer to Mr. D.'s wishes was ultimately influenced by a "belief in the rights of individuals to determine their own destinies." Yet, I might not have deferred to Mr. D.'s wishes, if he had without any explanation persisted in his refusal to undergo diagnostic tests. Before proceeding, I must draw attention to the fact that Siegler's account of his and the psychiatrist's interviews are devoid of any data as to why Mr. D. was so adamant in his refusal. I shall assume that Siegler and the psychiatrist were unable to elicit any information from Mr. D. about his reasons for refusing the tests. That assumption is crucial for what follows, for Siegler may have data on that issue which, if he had presented them in his article, might have led me to the same decision that he made.

Had Mr. D. been unwilling to give me his reasons for the refusal, I might have gone forward with the diagnostic tests. Since overruling a patient's choice is an awesome decision, I must both define the conditions in which a physician ought to consider taking such action and justify such exceptions to the rule of respecting patients' choices.

I would consider disobeying a patient's choice when two conditions have been met: One, the consequences on non-intervention pose grave risks to a patient's immediate physical condition *and*, two, the process of thinking about choices is so seriously impaired that neither physician nor patient seem to know what one or both wish to convey to the other.

With respect to the first condition, I would limit interferences with patients' choices to illnesses for which available diagnostic and therapeutic interventions have a reasonable chance of preventing death or predictable, serious, and irreversible physical injuries in instances when death or injury would occur within a relatively short period of time. (The emphasis on serious physical consequences seeks to balance the values of respect for self-determination and well-being. The emphasis on the time factor seeks to acknowledge that it can take time to clarify confusion and misconceptions. For example, time may not be available when, without intervention, death or injury are imminent.)

The first condition, however, is only a *necessary* one for intervention, it is *not decisive* by itself. Interference with patients' choices must also meet another test: The process of thinking about choices must be seriously impaired. It is this second condition that I want to address at greater length. In Chapter V, I observed that *both* physicians and patients are obligated to converse with one another in order to clarify their respective positions; that neither physician nor patient can easily repudiate that requirement, at least not the physician, and the patient only after he has made a good case for wishing to do so.

Before trying to justify why the overruling of patients' choices should be given serious consideration if these two conditions prevail, I want to say more about Mr. D. Had I encountered Mr. D., I would have told him that I was puzzled by his refusal to undergo the proposed diagnostic tests. I would have expressed to him my concern and confusion over my lack of understanding of what had led him to his decision, as well as my concern and fear of perhaps not having adequately conveyed to him why I thought that these tests were so essential to his well-being.

I would have impressed on him the necessity of our talking together. Indeed, I would have insisted on our talking together as long as time permitted in order to clarify our respective positions. I would have promised him that I had every intention of ultimately respecting his wishes, but that I could not make an absolute promise to do so, for it could turn out that the acuteness and seriousness of his condition might require an intervention prior to our having made ourselves understood to one another. I would have added that I expected this to be an unlikely outcome, but that it could happen. Throughout, I would have tried to convey to Mr. D. that my insistence on conversation was based on two concerns: to make sure that I had cleared up any of his misconceptions and confusion about the need for the diagnostic tests, and that he understood why I considered the performance of these tests so essential.

If in the midst of our talking together, Mr. D. had "turned away," and bid me to "leave [him] alone," I would not have left his bedside. Such conduct would have been tantamount to acting as "if I had not been there in the first place, as if I could be totally obliterated before [Mr. D.] succeeded in obliterating himself."[19] I would have felt impotent and experienced Mr. D. as all powerful. And I would have recalled what Burt had written in *Taking Care of Strangers* that such depictions of myself and him might have enraged me and made me turn away out of an unconscious wish to hurt him. At the same time, I might have overlooked that the patient too, appearances notwithstanding, was struggling with feelings of impotence out of "the intense stress [he was suffering] from the incapacitating experience of his illness." Thus, I would have stayed with him and renewed my invitation to talk with one another. Had he continued to decline the invitation, I would eventually have been forced to tell him that I might very well order the tests, place him on a respirator, and resuscitate him if he refused to talk with me. "There is too much that we both do not understand," I would have added, "and you must not hide behind silence."

I can only speculate about how my insistence to talk with Mr. D. might have affected him. It might have pierced his isolation and uncommunicativeness, and led him to express his concern and confusion over the proposed tests. Perhaps he viewed them as experimental rather than as a diagnostic necessity. After all, some patients are convinced that doctors at university hospitals like to conduct experiments on patients.[20] In this connection, it is important to note that Siegler learned only after Mr. D.'s death that "ten years earlier [Mr. D.] had left a hospital 'against medical advice' after first refusing to have a bone marrow examination." Since in the intervening years he had not been any worse off for his refusal, he might have wondered whether this test was not equally unnecessary now. Had he told me about this experience, perhaps I could have impressed on him that the two situations were not necessarily comparable. From there, we could have gone on to talk about his mistrust of doctors and the uncertainties of medicine. Who knows what else we might then have explored.

Moreover, Mr. D. clearly wished to be treated and *only* refused the performance of diagnostic tests. Something incomprehensible was at work here that begged for clarification. And if it could not be clarified, how could one judge the state of his autonomy? It seems that a conflict existed between his "autonomous" wish to be cured and his "autonomous" refusal to undergo diagnostic tests. Which deserved respect?

If on the basis of my nagging and unanswered questions I had intervened, I would not have done so because I thought his decision unwise, foolish or whatever, but because I had no idea whatever why he had decided what he did. I would have felt confused and been uncertain whether he was confused as well.

I find the case for intervention relatively easy to defend, if Mr. D. had persisted in his refusal to consent to the diagnostic tests without *any* explanation. It is more difficult to find an answer to a crucial question that an exception to the rule of respect for a patient's choice poses for the limits to such interventions: What could Mr. D. have told me that would have led me to bow to his decision? It is easy to answer this question at the other end of the continuum from patients' silence to communication. For example, if Mr. D. had been a Jehovah's Witness and refused the tests on religious grounds, I would still have talked with him but readily accepted his decision. Between the poles of utter silence about his reasons and expressions of deeply held personal beliefs that dictated his refusal, I would have listened to him, guided by a presumption in favor of respecting his decision; a presumption that could only be overcome by serious concerns on my part that we had not been able to clarify misconceptions, distortions and ignorance, and that I had not been able to impress on him that he mattered and was worthy of my time and effort.

Concerns over the impact of misconceptions and distortions on patients' choice loom large in my mind. Ruth and Alan Faden have written about a case in point. A 57-year-old woman had refused a hysterectomy for the treatment of cervical cancer on the ground that "she did not believe she had cancer. 'Anyone knows,' she said, 'that people with cancer are sick, feel bad and lose weight,' while she felt quite well.''[21] Arguments to the contrary were of no avail, until it was discovered that "the fact that her treating physician was black [had been] a major reason for her not believing that she had cancer. Discussions with another physician (who was white) and with her daughter resulted in a change in belief." Without sustained conversation her reasons for the initial refusal of a hysterectomy might never have been clarified and condemned her to an unnecessary death.

A personal experience raises the same issue. Some time ago, a group of pediatricians consulted me about a 15-year-old girl's refusal to undergo surgery for repair of a congenital heart defect. At age 5, she had been operated on for the same condition and for 10 years had enjoyed good health. She now was slowly decompensating again and, unless a second operation was performed, most likely would die within 5–10 years. That operation had a high mortality (up to 30 percent) but, if successful, promised complete recovery. She refused, not because of the surgical risks, but because of her fears over suffering "intolerable" postoperative pain. Her doctors were puzzled. They were prepared to respect a refusal based on fears over the high operative risks. Yet, this fact was of no concern to her. Instead, she had told them that she would have been quite willing to face death because, if successful, the operation would restore her to complete health. She based her refusal on her unwillingness to suffer postoperative pain. The doctors' promise to employ pain-relieving medication postoperatively in liberal amounts was of no avail; they were unable to convince her that they could keep her free from pain and suffering.

The pediatricians asked me what else they might do. During our discussion we talked about many things. For example, I raised the question of why they were willing to respect her refusal to undergo the operation, even though it was based on reasons that made no sense to them, and at the same time had been prepared to accept an affirmative response, even though they were troubled, but she seemed not, by the high risks of operative mortality? "Why," I asked, "was a 'yes' response not as suspect as a 'no' response?" My questions were met with a stunned and prolonged silence.

I was able to throw some light on the mystery of her concern over pain and suffering. As I listened to her doctors, I recalled painful memories, reported by patients in psychoanalytic treat-

ment, about childhood operations. These stories depicted the
sudden shift from happy childhood memories to painful ones
about hospitals and operations, memories of physical discomfort
that were augmented by psychic suffering and confusion over
what my patients had perceived as a "betrayal" by previously
caring parents who, they felt, had cruelly turned against them. I
wondered whether such excruciatingly painful, unconscious
memories might not have influenced her decision.

Since there was time before the operation had to be performed, I suggested that the doctors ask one of the hospital's psychiatric social workers to talk for a while with the young girl and
attempt to clarify the confusion between childhood memories
and current realities. Her story had a happy ending. She eventually agreed to the operation which proved successful.

In this instance, the availability of a person who could draw
on his professional experiences made the resolution of a puzzling
problem easier. Yet, even if I had not been there, a commitment
to conversation might have brought about the same result. In exploring her adamant belief that intolerable pain was inevitable,
she might have recalled her first operation and what she thought
had transpired then. Awareness of the confusion of past and
present could then have led to a clarification of its impact on her
initial decision. Both stories, I believe, reinforce the lessons to be
learned from Mr. D.'s case: the obligation to converse so that
misconceptions, confusion, fears, and ignorance can be clarified;
and the necessity not to accept prematurely patients' refusal to
engage in such conversations.

I appreciate the problem of occasional coercion that my prescription raises. While no principle can rule absolute, including
the principle of freedom of choice, exceptions to it must be most
narrowly circumscribed and justified. Let me add to what I have
already said about justifications. As my explorations in Chapter
V and the clinical examples of this chapter indicate, my views on
the need for an exception to unconditional respect for patient
choice is based on the concept of psychological autonomy. Respect for patients' vulnerability to ill-considered thoughts and
actions requires that they engage in conversation. Physicians
however, also have needs that deserve respect. In situations like
Mr. D.'s, their strong ethical commitment to caring for patients
can impose intolerable burdens on them. In these instances, doctors may never know whether they have explained themselves

satisfactorily to their patients. Doctors may then doubt whether they have taken the necessary time or made the necessary effort to make themselves understood. Such doubts can lead to nagging guilt feelings over having failed in one's professional obligations. Assuaging guilt-inducing doubts that may haunt physicians for a lifetime is another reason for my insistence on conversation.

Equally important is another consideration, highlighted by Mr. D.'s case. If all final authority is vested in patients, the danger is great that in situations of either a total refusal to give an account of one's reasons or an unwillingness to explore one's possible confusion—when the need for conversation is the greatest—doctors will wittingly and unwittingly give up on conversation and patients prematurely because they have been stripped of all power to stop even patients' most inexplicable self-destructive course. To protect doctors and, in turn, patients from such pernicious consequences supports the creation of a *rare* exception to the rule that doctors otherwise must obey: In case of disagreement, doctors and patients should either go their separate ways, or agree to provide and to receive care within the limits imposed by the patient.

Doctors, I believe, will rarely have to overrule patients' choices, *if* respect for conversation in preparation for choice were to become part of their ethical commitment. Patients would soon learn from their doctors' example that decision making in medicine can rarely be carried out in isolation, but only through mutual interaction. Thomas Aquinas appreciated this when he spoke of the need for "fraternal correction."[22] Or as Paul Tillich once put it, "humanity is attained by self-determination and by other-determination in mutual dependence."[23] Such insights will eventually make my limited exception to patient choice a relic of the past. Patients will learn to be less afraid to voice their reasons for refusal because they will be confident that such disclosures will only invite "fraternal correction" through conversation, but no more than that.

Summing up

It may be misplaced optimism to believe that when physician-patient conversations are conducted with a greater awareness of the biases, value judgments and different expectations that can affect recommendation and choice, it will generally lead to a reconciliation of any differing views between the parties: Either the physician will find it possible to agree with his patient's views, or the patient with the physician's, or some new solution will emerge out of their conversations. Conversation, however, will protect the integrity of the physician-patient relationship only if doctors are willing to confront and change their views of themselves as sole authority and of their patients as incompetent participants in decision making. Otherwise, manipulation and coercion will continue to rule their interactions. An inscription on a Greek temple comes to mind: "These are the duties of a physician: first . . . to heal his mind and to give assistance to himself before giving it to anyone (else). . . ."[24] These ancient duties command physicians to become aware of their own infirmities, to look at themselves before they attempt to help others. Only with a greater awareness of what transpires in their minds can physicians communicate meaningfully with their patients.

Dostoyevsky's Grand Inquisitor predicted that patients may not wish to assume the responsibilities engendered by that "terrible gift of freedom."[25] Throughout history, traditional patterns of physician-patient interaction seem to have made his prediction a self-fulfilling prophecy. If my views on psychological autonomy and its management have merit, however, it is not at all clear how valid his prediction has to remain.

My views impose new responsibilities for thinking about choices and choice. Even if these new responsibilities are accepted, decision making between physicians and patients will continue to remain beset by one nagging concern that can never be fully laid to rest: How much are their deliberations affected by irrational and unconscious influences for better or for worse? Yet the inevitable flaws in disclosure and consent from the perspective of psychological autonomy should not lead to the imposition or acceptance of silence instead.

A commitment to conversation creates new, formidable problems. It obligates physicians to acknowledge their uncertainties as well as the lack and incompleteness of collective and individual knowledge that stalk all professional practices. Doctors' reluctance, if not fear, of acknowledging medical uncertainty and ignorance has had an insufficiently appreciated influence on making the world of doctors and patients as silent as it is. It is to this problem I now turn.

VII

Acknowledging Uncertainty: The Confrontation of Knowledge and Ignorance

SINCE THE 1760's, whenever judges and counsel have dined at Sargeants' Inn Hall, the traditional toast to "the glorious memory of King William" has been followed by one to "the glorious uncertainty of the law."[1] The toast was first proposed in honor of Chief Justice Lord Mansfield, who had unsettled the legal community by overruling several long established legal precedents and by introducing a number of innovations in the practices of his court. The simultaneous celebration of authority and uncertainty was no accident. Nor was it a coincidence that uncertainty was celebrated when it would only engender momentary laughter before being drowned in ale and wine. This story from legal history serves as a reminder that the disquiet over uncertainty is not restricted to the medical profession.

With the exception of Renée Fox's pioneering studies,[2] the impact of uncertainty on professional practices has received little systematic attention from either lawyers or physicians. On reflection, this is not surprising. It is a fact of life that human beings find it difficult to maintain a consistent, self-conscious appreciation of the extent to which uncertainty accompanies them on their daily rounds and to integrate that uncertainty with whatever certainties inform their conduct. Physicians are not exempt from this human proclivity. They will acknowledge medicine's uncertainty once its presence is forced into conscious awareness, yet at the same time will continue to conduct their practices as if uncertainty did not exist.

The Gap between Theory and Practice

Medical knowledge is engulfed and infiltrated by uncertainty. In *Clinical Judgment* Alvan Feinstein has argued persuasively that

> [a]lthough anticoagulants, antibiotics, hypotensive agents, insulin, and steroids have been available for 15 to 40 years, many of their true effects on patients and diseases are unknown or equivocal. Clinicians are still uncertain about the best means of treatment for even such routine problems as a common cold, a sprained back, a fractured hip, a peptic ulcer, a stroke, a myocardial infarction, an obstetrical delivery, or an acute psychiatric depression. . . . At a time of potent drugs and formidable surgery, the exact effects of many therapeutic procedures are dubious and shrouded in dissension—often documented either by the unquantified data of 'experience' or by grandiose statistics whose mathematical formulations are so clinically naive that any significance is purely numerical rather than biologic.[3]

Yet the reality of medical uncertainty is generally brushed aside as doctors move from its theoretical contemplation to its clinical application in therapy and, even more so, in talking with their patients.

A conversation with a surgeon-friend illustrates this point. We first discussed at some length all the uncertainties that plague the treatment of breast cancer. We readily agreed on what was known, unknown, or conjectural about the varieties of therapeutic modalities offered to patients, such as surgery, radiation, and chemotherapy. I then asked how he would speak with a patient about the treatment of breast cancer. Since he had faced this difficult assignment only a few days earlier, he related to me this recent experience.

At the beginning of their encounter, he had briefly mentioned a number of available treatment alternatives. He added that he had done so without indicating that any of the alternatives to radical surgery deserved serious consideration. Instead, he had quickly impressed on his patient the need for submitting to this operation. I commented that he had given short shrift to other treatment approaches even though a few minutes earlier he had agreed with me that we still are so ignorant about which treatment is best. He seemed startled by my comment but responded with little hesitation that ours had been a theoretical discussion, of little relevance to practice. Moreover, he added emphatically that, in the light of present knowledge, radical surgery was the best treatment.

He then asked me what I might have done instead. I told him that I would have first clearly acknowledged our ignorance about which treatment is best. I would then have laid out all treatment modalities in considerable detail and discussed them with the patient. Eventually I would have made a recommendation but only after I had first elicited her preference *and* the reasons for her choice. Holding back for a while on giving her my recommendation would have served two purposes: one, to prevent her being pressured by my professional authority to accept my recommendation; and, two, to provide an additional opportunity to explore—if she had come to a decision unsupported either by the facts I had presented or her stated needs—why she had chosen that particular treatment. We would then have been better situated to clarify whether her decision was affected by a lack of understanding of what I had said or whether I had insufficiently appreciated her wishes, needs, and expectations. He responded that the patient we had been discussing—indeed, most of his patients—would not tolerate such explorations. Patients, he went on to say, do not have the capacity to understand such complex matters and, moreover, such conversations would cause them anxiety and intolerable pain. He also pointed to the specific danger of his patient choosing an inappropriate treatment because it seemed more pleasing in the short run, even if it were not in her best interest in the long run. I was particularly struck by his real concern about not causing his patient any pain. Yet, I also silently wondered whether he would have been equally, if not more, pained by having to converse with her about his certainties and uncertainties as to the choice of treatment.

In scrutinizing these two conversations, the surgeon's with his patient and mine with him, I was struck by a number of puzzling facts: First, he and I had been able to talk about the uncertainties surrounding the treatment of breast cancer without undue difficulty. We had agreed that nobody knew what is *the* one best treatment and we had also been able to discuss the specific indications and contraindications of various treatment modalities, their risks and benefits. While we could not do so with complete certainty, we conversed quite intelligibly, and without using many technical terms, about what was known and unknown about the likelihood of recurrence, the advantages and disadvantages of deferring adjuvant therapies, like chemotherapy, to a later time, and the impact of various treatments on longevity. In short, he and I could identify reasonably well the certainties and uncertainties inherent in the various approaches to the treatment of breast cancer. Yet, as he moved from theory to practice, my surgeon-friend—both in his conversation with me and with his patient—suddenly seemed to forget all that he had said about uncertainty. He spoke instead with considerable certainty, but no explanation, about the indication for only one form of treatment: radical mastectomy.

Second, when I challenged him about the discrepancy between his theoretical awareness of uncertainty and his certainty about what was best for his patient, he momentarily seemed surprised that I even would raise that issue. In response to my challenge, he did not address the tensions between theory and practice, but remarked without elaboration that they are separate domains which do not need to be bridged. It seemed to me, as he turned his attention to the clinical problem, that he had suddenly become unaware of the existence of uncertainty, that uncertainty had become split off and removed from consciousness.

Third, once challenged, my surgeon-friend spoke with conviction about how his patient could neither comprehend nor tolerate an exploration of the certainties and uncertainties inherent in the treatment of breast cancer. At the same time he admitted that he hardly knew this patient. He hastened to add, however, that his lack of familiarity with this particular patient was of little moment, because on the basis of considerable "clinical experience," he had learned that patients neither wish to nor can engage in such conversations. When I asked him to give me some examples of when he had tried to converse with patients about such matters, he paused for a while and then said that these incidents had happened so long ago that he could not clearly remember them. The certainty he had expressed about the choice of treatment seemed to be powerfully reinforced by convictions that related not to matters of medical knowledge but to his views about patients and the proper management of the physician-patient relationship.

In trying to make sense out of these observations, three problems that uncertainty of medical knowledge poses for physician-patient decision making deserve separate attention. One is engendered by the interrelationship between certainty and uncertainty inherent in medical knowledge itself. Uncertainty here raises the question: Is medicine sufficiently advanced so that doctors can be aware of, and distinguish between, opinions and recommendations based on certainty, uncertainty, or a mixture of both? The second problem is created by disclosures of uncertainties to patients. Disclosure of uncertainty here raises two questions: Can patients comprehend medicine's "esoteric" knowledge, in general, and its accompanying certainties and uncertainties, in particular? And is the impact on patients of such disclosures ultimately beneficial or detrimental? The third problem is created by the impact on physicians of a greater awareness of uncertainty. Awareness of uncertainty here raises the question: Would contemplation of medical uncertainties diminish physicians' effectiveness as healers? The fear is that doctors might become so obsessed by questions and doubts that they could no longer act with the necessary dispatch and conviction.

The Disregard of Uncertainty

Beyond these three specific problems, a more general problem requires attention. Recall that my surgeon-friend initially was not only quite conscious of the uncertainties inherent in the treatment of breast cancer but also could separate uncertainty from certainty reasonably well. Moreover, whenever he disregarded the problem of uncertainty of knowledge and was challenged, he became aware of it once again. Thus a closer scrutiny of our conversation suggests the influence of two modes of thought on what he said to me: He could be fully conscious of, or oblivious to, the uncertainties of medical knowledge. He was more conscious of uncertainty when he addressed theoretical issues and oblivious of uncertainty when he was preoccupied with practical concerns.

The mode of thought that ignores uncertainty found expression in his recounting of how much he had impressed on his patient the need for radical surgery. It is hard to tell, without inquiry, whether he had momentarily, and without awareness, repressed all his knowledge about uncertainty—that is, denied uncertainty—or whether he was aware of uncertainty and for other reasons decided not to consider it. For now I only wish to point to the fact that it is possible not only to deny uncertainty but also quickly and effectively to suppress the emergence of any thoughts about uncertainty out of a conviction that it is to be eschewed in the practice of medicine. The distinguishing characteristic of this mode of thought is that the physician will tell a false or incomplete story not only to his patient but to himself as well.

The mode of thought that consciously considers uncertainty found expression when my surgeon-friend, once challenged by me, became immediately aware of medicine's uncertainties but proceeded to offer a number of justifications for his personal and professional beliefs. At these times, he did not tell a false story to himself, but felt, based on his "clinical experience" acquired during training and practice, that patients needed to be told a false or incomplete story. It is important to distinguish between these two modes of thought, because denial and habitual suppression of uncertainty make significant information unavailable to physicians themselves; even if they want to, they cannot impart such information to patients. Keeping uncertainty to oneself for other reasons, on the other hand, does not create this problem. Moreover, the reasons for withholding information about uncertainty may point up complex problems about the practice of medicine that deserve examination in their own right.

Our conversation also illustrates that uncertainty of medical knowledge itself is not at issue. To be sure, our conversation would have proceeded along different lines if medicine were not beset by pervasive uncertainties. One may wish it to be otherwise but this does not change the fact that uncertainty of knowledge will for a long time remain an essential characteristic of the practice of medicine. In fact, my surgeon-friend and I were able to talk comfortably and intelligibly about certainty and uncertainty. He only disregarded uncertainty when he was speaking about or to the patient. The actual or intrapsychic presence of the patient might have made him shift from one mode of thought to the other. In the presence of his patient his awareness of uncertainty became compromised, which precluded contemplation of the idea of acknowledging uncertainty to her. Thus the problem posed by uncertainty of knowledge for mutual decision making is how to keep the existence of uncertainty clearly in mind and not replace it by certainty whenever one moves from theoretical to practical considerations. Put another way, the problem is not uncertainty of medical knowledge but the capacity to remain aware of, and the willingness to acknowledge, uncertainty.

The defenses that physicians employ against an awareness of uncertainty have been well described by Renée Fox, who has made important contributions to the study of medical uncertainty. She identified "three basic types of uncertainty" that isolate particular stresses that affect physicians in the conduct of their work:

> The first results from incomplete or imperfect mastery of available knowledge. No one can have at his command all skills and all knowledge of the lore of medicine. The second depends upon limitations in current medical knowledge. There are innumerable questions to which no physician, however well trained, can as yet provide answers. A third source of uncertainty derives from the first two. This consists of difficulty in distinguishing between personal ignorance or ineptitude and the limitations of present medical knowledge.[4]

Fox emphasized the stresses caused by deficiencies in individual and collective professional knowledge, as well as by the difficulty of making clear distinctions between these two sets of deficiencies.

In her detailed study of doctors and patients on "Ward-F Second," a metabolic research unit, Fox documented the pervasive presence of uncertainty as a third party.[5] The doctors who worked on this ward were deeply committed to getting the better of uncertainty and they persevered despite many failures and the considerable stress that their dual obligations as investigators and clinicians imposed on them. Since the stresses were quite noticeable, Fox became intrigued to learn more about how the doctors coped with the stresses of uncertainty. She identified some of the defenses physicians employed against uncertainty—the "counterphobic impious grim joking . . . to come to terms with the most stressful aspects of their situation" and "the game of chance . . . the wagering behavior in which they engage" when predictions were hazardous. She emphasized that they devised "nonempirical or magical techniques to 'enable them to carry out their . . . tasks with confidence and poise.' "

The physicians on Ward-F Second were greatly troubled that their combined investigative and therapeutic interventions might expose their patients to harm. The doctors were aware of the significant contributions that uncertainty of knowledge made to the risks of harm, and they were able not only to talk with one another about uncertainty but also to identify, often with considerable specificity, what was known, unknown, and conjectural about their proposed interventions and their potentially harmful consequences. The defenses they employed were not directed against an awareness of the uncertainties of medical knowledge. Instead, they were directed against a fuller awareness of concerns about the impact of their activities on their personal and professional values and on their patients' well-being. The defenses allowed them to deny or at least moderate their concerns sufficiently so that they could continue to carry out their tasks with "confidence and poise."

The defenses that the doctors employed contributed to their not giving a great deal of thought to sharing their *specific* uncertainties about particular interventions with their patients. Fox's data bear testimony to the physicians' wish both to treat their patients as "colleagues" by making it initially clear to them that they were both patients and research subjects, and not to treat their patients as "colleagues" in their day-to-day encounters by failing to acknowledge to them their uncertainties in a great many specific instances. The defenses the physicians employed against their concerns about what they were doing to themselves and their patients, which led to their not acknowledging their uncertainties to patients, were reinforced by traditional attitudes of not asking patients to share the burdens of decision. "Like all patients," Fox noted, "the men of Ward-F Second were expected to entrust themselves to the physicians responsible for their care; to undergo the procedures that these physicians felt were necessary for the diagnosis and treatment of their conditions; to take the medications which had been prescribed for them; and, in general, to 'follow the doctors' orders.' "

The failure to acknowledge uncertainty could have resulted from a denial of uncertainty, from traditional ideas about the ethical conduct of physicians toward patients which can exist side by side with an awareness of uncertainty, or from habitual thoughts about the proper exercise of one's professional responsibilities which quickly suppress any budding awareness of uncertainty. The difficulty of making such distinctions has led me to encompass all three under the term *disregard of uncertainty*. The important lesson to be learned from Fox's study, as is equally true for the conversation with my surgeon-friend, is how pervasive the disregard of uncertainty becomes whenever uncertainty ceases to be merely theoretical and impinges on "the stressful aspects of [doctor's] situation" in actual clinical encounters. Fox's observations compellingly illustrate the difficulties of coping with uncertainty, if by coping is meant "struggling with, contending with," and not trying to put it out of mind. Thus, while the very existence of uncertainty imposes burdens on physicians, the greater burden is the obligation to keep these uncertainties in mind and to acknowledge them to patients.

Another example, provided by George Crile, Jr., illustrates a more total denial of uncertainty, caused by psychological forces that are deeply embedded in the unconscious and difficult to overcome. The existence of such defensive operations define some of the limits of human capacities to become aware of uncertainty. These limits must be accepted, although the restrictions they impose on awareness can be moderated. Crile wrote that his father, George Crile, Sr., a renowned surgeon of the early twentieth century under whom he trained, "*never* did a radical mastectomy."[6] Instead, his father always employed a less mutilating surgical procedure. George Crile, Jr. continued, "[d]uring my residency at the Cleveland Clinic, I was also exposed to the influence of Dr. Tom Jones, who *always* did a radical mastectomy. Being a rebellious child, I discounted my father's ideas, adopted the Jones technique, and for seventeen years I performed only radical mastectomies." Now, however, Crile concluded, "[c]onventional radical mastectomies are not done" at the Cleveland Clinic.

Having been trained by his father and Jones, Crile was aware of the uncertainties that surrounded the proper treatment of breast cancer, but he was compelled to deny uncertainty and substitute an uncompromising certainty in its place for powerful personal reasons. His conversion raises many questions. In now following his father, has he merely become a compliant child? How can he know? Or, put differently, to what extent can he demand that patients trust him implicitly since he was so readily affected by oedipal conflicts, which he fought out over the bodies of countless Jocastas? Indeed, to what extent do many surgeons, trained by other illustrious "fathers," replicate this struggle by performing only procedures prescribed by their elders' paternal authority, to which they submit passively because they have not sufficiently resolved their conflicts with their biological fathers? I enlist these psychological considerations both to emphasize how these and other powerful forces can defeat an awareness of uncertainty, and to encourage a more self-conscious and reflective recognition of the constant presence of uncertainty in medical practice. Such heightened awareness may alert physicians to the fact that something may be amiss whenever single-mindedness dominates their therapeutic interventions.

The denial of uncertainty, the proclivity to substitute certainty for uncertainty, is one of the most remarkable human psychological traits. It is both adaptive and maladaptive, and therefore both guides and misguides. In one of his earlier works, *The Interpretation of Dreams*, Freud observed how, immediately upon awakening, the dreamer distorts the senselessness of his dream as dreamt by giving it a coherence that it did not possess. He wrote:

> [I]t is our normal thinking that . . . approaches the content of dreams with a demand that it must be intelligible. . . .
>
> *   *   *
>
> It is the nature of our waking thought to establish order in material of that kind, to set up relations in it and to make it conform to our expectations of an intelligible whole. . . . An adept in sleight of hand can trick us by relying upon this intellectual habit of ours. In our efforts at making an intelligible pattern of the sense-impressions that are offered to us, we often fall into the strangest errors or even falsify the truth about the material before us.[7]

Similarly, other studies have demonstrated how witnesses at scenes of accidents unwittingly fill in their incomplete perceptions and recollections with "data" that will give coherence to both their certainties and uncertainties about what has transpired.

Human beings' defensive and adaptive needs to make both their internal and external worlds intelligible, to shun incomprehensibility, doubt, and uncertainty, are formidable. In dreams, it is the simultaneous presence of contradictory, "absurd" and irrational unconscious thoughts and of more accustomed rational thoughts—all of which make up the content of dreams—that is largely denied. Witnesses to accidents defend against the faulty nature of their external sense perceptions. Both examples illustrate the pervasive and fateful human need to remain in control over one's internal and external worlds by seemingly understanding them, even at the expense of falsifying the data.

Physicians' denial of awareness of uncertainty serves similar purposes: it makes matters seem clearer, more understandable, and more certain than they are; it makes action possible. There are limits to living with uncertainty. It can paralyze action. This is particularly true, as John Dewey noted, in practical affairs, as in the practice of medicine, where decisions must be made. He chided his fellow-philosophers on their futile quest for certainty to obtain relief from the tremendous insecurities of human existence. He argued that "the idea of any complete synthesis of knowledge upon an intellectual basis" is an impossible quest. "Man has never had such a varied body of knowledge in his possession before, and probably never before has been so uncertain and so perplexed as to what his knowledge means, what it points to in action and in consequences."[8] This insight did not suggest to Dewey an abandonment of the quest for greater certainty. He concluded instead that it is "the vital office of present philosophy . . . to search out and disclose the obstructions; to criticize the habits of mind which stand in the way [of] the development of an [integrated] system of thought." This objective, too, has its limits because of the constant admixture of certainty and uncertainty. Nevertheless, it should be the "vital office" of scientific medicine to develop systems of thought and action that will permit physicians to account more fully for both the certainties and uncertainties that shape their practices. To achieve such an objective will not prove easy, for formidable obstacles, to which I now turn, impede the awareness and acknowledgment of uncertainty in the practice of medicine.

A History of Uncertainty:
The Treatment of Breast Cancer

The history of the treatment of breast cancer illustrates some of the problems that uncertainty about medical knowledge has posed for decision making between physicians and patients throughout the ages. I shall present its early history briefly in order to make the point that, until recently, physicians had to profess certainty about the treatment of breast cancer because they possessed neither the experimental nor the intellectual tools to distinguish between certainty and uncertainty. Every proposed treatment, however valuable or silly, found its enthusiastic adherents. If it eventually fell into disrepute because of lack of any success, it was quickly replaced by another method, touted with equal certainty. I shall then discuss two episodes from modern history to explore the impact of scientific thought and experimentation on the problem of awareness and acknowledgment of uncertainty. With physicians' increasing intellectual and scientific capacities to distinguish between certainty and uncertainty in knowledge, it is no longer so much uncertainty that plagues physician-patient decision making, but the disregard of uncertainty.

Pre-Modern Treatments of Breast Cancer

Breast cancer was probably known to the ancient Egyptians and surely was known to the Greeks, who treated it by surgery, caustic agents and a variety of medicines—mineral, vegetable, and animal.[9] Physicians employed many treatment modalities throughout the ages—bleeding, dieting, purging, using lead plates to compress the tumor, and applying goat dung, with each treatment being advocated in the belief that it was the best. William Clowes, physician to Queen Elizabeth I, resorted to exorcism, the laying on of royal hands, a venerable tradition dating back to Edward the Confessor whose "royal touch" was considered curative. With a queen on the throne, it is not surprising that Clowes expected that her hands would prove particularly curative for her suffering sisters. Yet, surgery seems always to have been the predominant mode of treatment, when treatment was attempted at all. Already in medieval times, "extensive and sweeping removals" of breast cancers were advocated, and many of the leading surgeons, then and into the twentieth century, chastised their colleagues for being too timid by leaving diseased tissue behind in the fond hope that it would "not grow, because it [was] such a little bit."[10] In different ages, either therapeutic pessimism or therapeutic optimism swayed doctors' attitudes toward treatment. Optimism was fueled, as it is today, by the belief that in the presence of deadly disease it is the physician's duty boldly to try everything.

Any uncertainties that physicians entertained about their favorite treatment modalities became imperceptibly blended with the certainty that they finally had discovered a cure. Convictions about the value of their remedies found additional support in various philosophical theories that guided their treatments, such as theories about the influence on disease of "temperaments" or "humours" (blood, phlegm, yellow bile and black bile). To say that physicians in these early days disregarded uncertainty makes little sense. They did not understand how and whether their treatments really worked. Conflicting claims could not be subjected to experimental verifications and thus, by and large treatment had to remain a matter of faith in the curative power of individual physicians. Careful observations of individual patients by a handful of physicians provided some insights about outcome, but these were undermined by unsupported claims of cure advanced by most practicing physicians.

Modern Treatments: Radical Mastectomy

The modern approach to treatment of breast cancer can be divided into two phases. The first began in the late 1860's, when radical surgery emerged as the treatment of choice and, until most recently, was accepted without question by the majority of physicians. Even though William S. Halsted was not the first to propose it, his surgical technique—the en bloc removal of the entire breast, the underlying chest muscles, and the lymph nodes in the armpit—a treatment which his zeal brought to preeminence, deservedly bears his name. In the United States, it was adopted by the majority of practicing surgeons. His 1894 paper, optimistically entitled, "The Results of Operations for the Cure of Cancer of the Breast Performed at The Johns Hopkins Hospital from June, 1889 to January, 1894," electrified the medical community and quickly transformed the prevailing pessimism about treatment into optimism.[11]

How could it have been otherwise? The one-sentence opening paragraph of Halsted's paper read: "In 50 cases operated upon by what we call the complete method we have been able to trace only three local recurrences." This most remarkable achievement, never duplicated, led Halsted to conclude his paper by observing dispassionately that he could understand why, until then, many physicians had despaired of breast cancer's treatability and thus had not referred their patients to surgeons. But he went on to assert that from now on matters were different: "Now we can state *positively* that cancer of the breast is a curable disease if operated upon properly and in time. I cannot emphasize too strongly the fact that internal metastases occur very early in cancer of the breast, and this is an additional reason for not losing a day in discussing the propriety of an operation."

We now know, or think we know, that Halsted's operation was based on the false premise that breast cancer spreads from its original focus to outlying areas in an uninterrupted fashion. His reliance on that premise dictated only one cure: the en bloc removal of all tissue to which the cancer might have spread. Since the extent of microscopic involvement could not be fully ascertained by the surgeon's naked eyes, a considerable amount of healthy-looking tissue also had to be resected. To Halsted and his followers mutilation was an unfortunate and inevitable consequence. But a life was at stake.

Halsted's views found immediate and wide acceptance. Only occasionally were some mild reservations raised. For example, in 1898, while commenting on one of Halsted's papers, Rudolph Matas expressed his disappointment with the results of this radical procedure: "[S]ince 1894 I have operated upon a series of cases by the [Halsted] methods, and yet I have against my record 67.7 percent of failures, whereas in the preceding series of 10 cases, treated by less severe methods, I have had 40 percent recoveries, with only 33 percent total failures."[12] Despite his own findings, Matas hastened to add his appreciation of "the merit of the more extensive [Halsted] operation," and he concluded "that whatever the fallacies that underlie the so-called radical operation for cancer of the breast, as a curative procedure, we are under lasting obligations to Dr. Halsted for the suggestion and demonstration of an operation which synthesizes in itself all the recourses that modern surgery can bring to bear against this most formidable disease."

Note the doubts as well as the surrender. There were other surgeons who soon thereafter expressed misgivings about the value of radical surgery over less extensive surgical procedures.

The weight of Halsted's authority, however, was so great that a number of surgeons experienced difficulties in getting papers published that disputed his claims.[13] Others did not even dare to submit their contrary results. Fifty years had to elapse before serious reservations about Halsted's operation were with increasing insistence raised by distinguished members of the medical profession.

On the basis of the most limited data, Halsted's sweeping claims about the defeat of an ancient foe were accepted by the medical community. It is true that Halsted published his results at a time when medical science was still in its infancy; however, the scientific method had already begun to exert its influence over the practice of medicine. Academic physicians in particular had become sensitized to the need not only to subject innovative treatments to carefully controlled studies but also to await confirmation of their findings by other investigators. Yet, Halsted's claims were accepted despite that fact that by that time physicians were well aware that the history of medical practices was studded with instances of harm done to patients in the darkness of deeply held, unquestioned professional beliefs. For example, the story of Benjamin Rush, a signer of the Declaration of Independence and an eminent physician of his time, was well known. Convinced of the efficacy of bloodletting and purges for the treatment of a great many medical maladies, Rush employed them with abandon during the plague epidemic, killing patients who would have survived if left untreated. Rush lived prior to the modern scientific era, but Halsted was practicing in a different age. In saying this, I do not question Halsted's considerable accomplishments. I only wish to highlight his certainty about the correctness of his recommendations. Recall that he wrote, after a long history of dismal failure to cure breast cancer, "we can state positively that cancer of the breast is a curable disease."

This episode from the age of Halsted is a not uncommon example of how hard it is for human beings to live with doubt and uncertainty and of their proclivity to embrace certainty instead. The widespread and enthusiastic acceptance of Halsted's findings by most of his fellow physicians, even after repeated failures to cure breast cancer by radical mastectomy, demonstrates how readily any awareness of uncertainty succumbs to venerable authority and orthodoxy. These powerful defenses against awareness of uncertainty continue to rule professional practices. Sir

Geoffrey Keynes appreciated the commanding influence of orthodoxy and authority on professional practice. In a remarkable paper, "Carcinoma of the Breast—The Unorthodox Views" (1954), he used words rarely spoken by a surgeon:

> Orthodoxy in surgery is like orthodoxy in other departments of the mind—it starts as a tentative belief in some particular course of action, but later begins almost to challenge comparison with a religion. It comes to be held as a passionate belief in the absolute rightness of that particular view. A dissentient view is regarded as a criminal subversion of the truth, and the holder is sometimes exposed to slander and abuse. . . . None of us have been burnt at the stake, but feelings have run pretty high. . . .[14]

His paper was not published, as it should have been, in *The Lancet*, but in a secondary medical journal. I do not know whether he had dared to submit it to *The Lancet*'s editors and whether they had rejected it. In his day the controversy over the proper treatment of breast cancer was treated by polite silence. This is less true now. The passions it can evoke are testified to by the recent debate between two distinguished surgeons, Thomas J. Anglem of Boston and George Crile, Jr. of Cleveland.[15] They not only disagreed vehemently on the respective merits of radical against less extensive surgery, but one also felt compelled to call the other "almost paranoid." Since they could not question each other's professional credentials, one tried to question the other's rationality.

To return to Halsted, he practiced at a turning point in medical history. Science had just begun to influence ancient medical practices that relied on keen clinical observation and intuition in order to sort out the useless from the useful. Intuition without systematic observations grounded in a scientific methodology, however, can be treacherous. Even when it is not treacherous, recourse to clinical intuition makes it well-nigh impossible to evaluate the competing and often contradictory claims of success and failure advanced by practitioners. Moreover, problems of evaluation are compounded by difficulties in distinguishing the effects produced by physicians' "curative" interventions from those produced by nature's self-healing capacities and from those produced by the therapeutic presence of the healer, irrespective of his physical interventions. While the advent of modern science allowed physicians to cope better with all these problems,

Halsted should serve as a reminder that orthodoxy and authority are powerful forces that tend to obliterate awareness of uncertainty; they do not easily bow to the contrary claims of science: that in the search for truth, professionals must constantly scrutinize their certainties against the uncertainties of existing medical knowledge.

Lewis Thomas, a physician deeply committed to the practice of scientific medicine, has called attention to physicians' increasing capacity in the light of modern science to be more aware of their ignorance and uncertainty:

> The only solid piece of scientific truth about which I feel totally confident is that we are profoundly ignorant about nature. Indeed, I regard this as the major discovery of the past hundred years of biology. . . . It is this sudden confrontation with the depth and scope of ignorance that represents the most significant contribution of twentieth-century science to the human intellect. *We are, at last, facing up to it.* In earlier times, we either pretended to understand how things worked or ignored the problem or simply made up stories to fill the gaps.[16]

Thomas may be too optimistic in his belief that professionals now do not make ''up stories to fill the gaps.'' At least, too few face up to medicine's uncertainty. But I agree that in today's age of science the means for facing up to our ignorance exist as they never did before. Yet it is precisely this potential for greater clarity of what is known and unknown that has not been sufficiently heeded in medical practice in general, and in decision making between physicians and patients in particular.

Physicians do not have to disregard uncertainty so thoroughly. Thomas, aware of both the pitfalls and the potentialities of science, points doctors in the right direction:

> . . . The scientific method is guesswork, the making up of stories. The difference between this and other imaginative works of the human mind is that science is then obliged to find out whether the guesses are correct, the stories true. Curiosity drives the enterprise, and the open acknowledgment of ignorance. [W]e know very little about nature and we understand even less.
>
> Starting with ourselves, and the life immediately around us, we have lots of homework to do, lots of pride to swallow, lots more ignorance to face, some of it only sensed out of the corner of the eye. . . .[17]

An appreciation of medicine's vast ignorance could make physicians more cautious about claims to have found *the* answer to the treatment of any disease, particularly during the early stages of the discovery of a new and "promising" therapy. Assuming that pride can be swallowed, such an appreciation also permits making distinctions between ignorance and knowledge. A look at a second, more recent episode in the treatment of breast cancer may clarify what I have in mind.

Modern Treatments: Beyond Radical Mastectomy

In the early 1930's, doubts began to be raised about the premise that breast cancer spreads by continuous, centrifugal permeation. Injection studies with contrast media had led to inferences that the spread of breast cancer is often discontinuous in space, that it is disseminated to outlying lymph nodes by cancer emboli and to other areas by way of blood channels. These findings were largely disregarded by practicing surgeons, however. Moreover, other studies suggested that improvements in cure rates were more a function of earlier detection than of the extensiveness of the surgical procedures employed. (It was soon learned, however, that early detection was not *the* answer either.) These and other considerations moved a few surgeons, like Sir Geoffrey Keynes of England and Oliver Cope and George Crile, Jr. of the United States, to abandon radical surgical treatments.

Their decision was aided by advances in radiation therapy which led them to combine conservative surgery with radiation treatment. Yet for a long time their voices were crying in a hostile wilderness in which mutilating surgery continued to be inflicted on countless women. Indeed, their colleagues often shunned and severely censured them for their unorthodox views.[18] More important, the two groups divided into hostile camps, as the unusually acrimonious debates, carried on in scientific journals between Anglem, an advocate of radical surgery, and Crile, a champion of more conservative treatment, so clearly demonstrate.[19] Anglem and Crile bombarded each other with scientific data, often interpreting the same scientific studies differently, and they unwaveringly clung to the correctness of their respective positions. Rabid convictions do not lend themselves to the admission of uncertainty. Thus it made little difference to either of them that Bernard Fisher, another authority on breast cancer, had asserted, and I believe correctly, that we simply do not know which treatment is best.[20] Why his conclusion, so true in theory, remains so unacceptable in practice, even today, requires explanation.

If one contemplates the current status of the treatment of breast cancer, it becomes apparent that one has to think about the problem of uncertainty of medical knowledge in more discriminating ways. Since the turn of this century, we have acquired bits and pieces of knowledge about the vagaries of breast cancer and its response to treatment,[21] as well as the intellectual and experimental tools to discriminate better between what we know, what is still conjectural, and what is still shrouded in ignorance. For example, in the 1980's we think we know that, from its beginnings, breast cancer is generally a systematic disease and that complex, as yet poorly understood host-tumor interactions affect the progression of the disease. We also seem to know that even with very early discovery and treatment, some breast cancers will lead to death sooner or later, and that others respond favorably even when treated after considerable delay. We also seem to know that surgery, from its most limited to its most extensive varieties, as well as radiation therapy, chemotherapy, hormone therapy, and immunotherapy in various combinations and permutations of their own, and with surgery have therapeutic impact. Moreover, we seem to know that biological and genetic factors have a considerable impact on breast cancer control and cure, and that therefore any of these treatments can be detrimental, most likely by interfering with delicate tumor-host balances. Despite all these and other problems, we also seem to know that some treatment is better than none.

What we do not know, however, is which treatment is best. Most likely any or all of these theories of cure will be modified or discarded over time. They attest to our vast ignorance about the big picture but they also attest to our knowing a great many significant bits and pieces about the treatment of breast cancer.

Of importance to decision making between physician and patient is the fact that, if they are so inclined, physicians now can make clearer distinctions between what they know and do not know. Thus, they can offer patients a variety of treatment options based on pieces of evidence from available clinical data. *There is no certainty about the available knowledge, but its uncertainty can be specified.* This crucial point holds true for the treatment not only of breast cancer but for many other diseases as well.

Training for Certainty

Yet if one surveys the medical scene, once one leaves the arena of laboratory and clinical experimentation, there is little evidence that physicians more consciously take uncertainty into account either in their self-reflections or in their interactions with patients. The avoidance of uncertainty is reinforced by the ways in which future physicians are socialized during their medical and postgraduate education and by the contemporary organizational structure of medicine. The *training for certainty* begins in medical schools, and specialization also reinforces the quest for certainty. I would like to explore in somewhat greater detail doctors' flight from uncertainty as it emerges in their training and socialization, in the profession's demand for conformity—a variant of orthodoxy and authority—and in the pursuit of specialization. Without reform of these institutional practices, little will change.

The socialization of physicians reinforces the universal human tendency to turn away from uncertainty. I shall base my discussion of the socialization of medical students on Fox's seminal paper, "Training for Uncertainty."[22] Her intensive observations of Cornell medical students during their progression from the first to the fourth year led her to the conclusion that future physicians are trained for coping with uncertainty. I interpret her observations differently. Before proceeding, let me acknowledge my great debt for her exquisite observations, without which a different reading would have been impossible.

In a recent paper, Fox succinctly summarized the conclusions she had reached years earlier about Cornell medical students' "training for uncertainty":

> Some of the collective ways of coming to terms with uncertainty that medical students progressively developed were junior versions of the coping mechanisms that the physicians of Ward F-Second employed. These mechanisms included achieving as much cognitive command of the situation as possible, through the acquisition of greater medical knowledge and technical skill, and the increasing mastery of the probability-reasoning logic with which modern med-

icine approaches the uncertainties of differential diagnosis, treatment decisions, and prognosis-setting. . . . Students gradually evolved what they referred to as a more "affirmative attitude" toward medical uncertainty. They became more able to accept uncertainty as inherent in medicine, to sort out their own limitations from those of the field, meet uncertainty with candor, and to take a "positive, philosophy-of-doubting" approach. In clinical situations, they were more prone to feel and display sufficient "certitude" to make decisions and reassure patients. At the same time, the fact that students made numerous jokes about uncertainty, like Ward F-Second's physicians, indicated that this continued to be a source of stress.[23]

Fox is correct that during medical students' preclinical education, which spans the first two years of medical school, students are made aware of the existence of uncertainty.[24] Yet a close look at her observations suggests that even at that time, they are led to attribute much of their uncertainty not to its inevitable presence or to its pervasiveness but to their lack of training, to not having as "yet developed the discrimination and judgment of a skilled diagnostician." Moreover, they are already then being taught passively "to tolerate," in the sense of to endure and to suffer, uncertainty. They are not taught how to confront the reality and pain of uncertainty actively and systematically. They are promised instead that the pains of uncertainty will be mitigated, that "cognitive learning and a greater sense of certainty go hand in hand." To be sure, as time goes on, medical students feel more comfortable to doubt, to be unsure, but Fox's data are silent on how students learn to address "inevitable" and "legitimate" uncertainty and make effective use of their doubts in thought and action. The data speak much more to how students learn and acquire habits of certainty.

Fox herself noted that "[o]ne gains the impression that students are more uncertain during the first part of the third year than they were before, but that they become less uncertain than before during the later part of the third year." She gives many reasons for this progression from uncertainty to certainty: the closeness of their relationship to the clinical faculty, whose perceived self-assurance fosters, rather than casts doubt on, students' quest for certainty; the demand by their elders that students commit themselves to one or the other of their tentative judgments; and, most tellingly, the fear of criticism from their instructors whenever they display "too great [an] unsureness." They are exhorted by their teachers to be "firm and to take a position" and not to remain in doubt, for that will only impair their effectiveness vis-à-vis patients. Thus, by the end of the fourth year, students find "ways of adjusting to their *remaining* uncertainties; of meeting [their] uncertainty with greater confidence and equipoise."

By the fourth year, according to Fox's observations, 97% of Cornell medical students were "quite sure" or "fairly sure" that they could deal with problems of uncertainty. This astounding figure is most telling testimony to the training for certainty and control, rather than for uncertainty in medical education. John C. Whitehorn has deplored this progression, particularly since the ethos of science dictates otherwise:

> The educational programs generally experienced by the physicians of the past few generations have tended (without our intending it) to inculcate an expectation of certainty of knowledge and a phobic aversion for and intolerance of *uncertainty*, and the worst offenders have been teachers of science. This has been an error—a stultifying error. To inculcate the expectation of certainty of knowledge is a serious betrayal of the essence of the scientific movement. . . .[25]

To become true "specialists in uncertainty," a felicitous term coined by Fox,[26] requires a different education. In the light of the uncertainties that pervade medical practice, such an education must teach students not only how to live with failure but also how to remain more aware of uncertainty, how to proceed in the face of uncertainty, and how to decide which uncertainties to share with patients. Students must learn, as James B. Conant put it, that "[t]here are areas of experience where we know that uncertainty is the certainty."[27]

Conformity and Orthodoxy

Conformity and orthodoxy, playing the game according to the tenets of the group to which students wish to belong, are encouraged in medical, as in all professional, education; they further compromise awareness of uncertainty. I recall that during my first year at medical school we were one day instructed by the faculty of one distinguished university hospital that anticoagulant therapy was the treatment of choice for threatening pulmonary embolization and that any other therapy constituted unprofessional conduct, while at another equally distinguished hospital, we were informed that the only correct treatment was the surgical ligation of the inflamed veins. One could view such an exposure to controversy as training for uncertainty. I believe it is not. In neither hospital were we exposed to the complexities of decision making in the light of each hospital's successes and failures with this treatment as contrasted with alternative treatments; nor were we encouraged to keep an open mind. In both we were educated for dogmatic certainty, for adopting one school of thought or the other, and for playing the game according to the venerable, though contradictory, rules that each institution sought to impose on its staff, students, and patients.

Kathleen Knafl and Gary Burkett described similar events in the training of orthopedic residents.[28] For example, a not unusual controversy over the indications for subjecting a 13 month-old girl to a leg-lengthening procedure led to the following stand-off. A fourth year resident, quoting from the scientific literature that favored one particular approach, was interrupted by the attending surgeon: "I know that's what he says, but that's *not the way we do it here.*" Then another attending surgeon interjected, "[t]hat's *the way some of us do it!*" Again, this is not an example of teaching uncertainty; rather, it is an illustration of the rejection of scientific controversy in favor of personal preferences, of teaching conformity to one point of view or another. It was done by an appeal to clinical judgment and clinical experience. However important they are in their own right, clinical judgment and the adoption of one school of thought harbor their own built-in dangers. They constitute effective defenses against uncertainty. As Donald Light, Jr. observed:

> Clinical judgment and emphasizing technique redefine competence and mistakes in terms of technique, . . . But good technique in turn rests with the clinical judgment of the professional, which is essentially individual judgment. Thus in gaining control over their work by acquiring a treatment philosophy and exercising individual judgment without question, professionals run the danger of gaining too much control over the uncertainties of their work by becoming insensitive to complexities in diagnosis, treatment, and client relations.[29]

The assertion of clinical wisdom, based on personal experience, is difficult to refute; it can only be arbitrarily accepted or arbitrarily rejected.

Little seems to have changed with regard to "training for uncertainty" since Fox's studies and my experiences as a medical student. A few years ago in a seminar at the Yale Law School a young surgeon who had recently completed his training with a renowned surgeon, one of the most uncompromising advocates of radical breast surgery, joined my class of law students. During our discussion of a great many medical articles on the controversy over the treatment of breast cancer, he was unusually quiet. I finally turned to him and invited his comments. In an uncharacteristic outburst of temper, he pounded the table and practically shouted, "Anything but radical mastectomy is criminal conduct!" Subsequently, though still firmly committed to his views, he apologized for his "unpardonable" behavior. I thanked him because he had provided me and my students with a rare opportunity to experience the relentless power of deeply held personal and professional beliefs. Such orthodoxy will always remain a foe of an awareness and acknowledgment of uncertainty. As Thomas Kuhn has documented in his book, *The Structure of Scientific Revolutions*, shifts in paradigms may overturn orthodoxy, but only to clear the way for the establishment of a new orthodoxy.[30] One can only acknowledge this dynamic phenomenon and resist its excesses as best one can.

Specialization

In addition to the pressures of socialization and conformity, specialization, so prevalent in contemporary medical practice, contributes in its own way to the flight from uncertainty. Although specialization is to begin with an adaptive response to the vastness of medical knowledge, which no practitioner can master in its entirety, and, thus, ostensibly is an attempt to cope better with some forms of uncertainty, it paradoxically makes a significant contribution of its own to a spurious sense of certainty. Specialization tends to narrow diagnostic vision and to foster beliefs in the superior effectiveness of treatments prescribed by one's own specialty. This effect of specialization is reflected in the contemporary treatment of most diseases. Again, breast cancer provides a good illustration. Surgeons, radiation therapists and chemotherapists are in vehement disagreement over the respective merits of their treatments, usually without sufficiently doubting the effectiveness of their own treatment or respecting their competitors' treatment. As a consequence, a chance first encounter by a patient with one or another therapist may influence the treatment ultimately "chosen," regardless of what the patient might have chosen if provided with other options that are equally approved medically.

The public, and professionals as well, need to become more aware of the fact that many disparate groups now live under medicine's tent. Contemporary medicine is not a unitary profession but a federation of professions with differing ideologies and senses of mission. This diversification has changed medical practices. At the turn of the century, when allopathic physicians were first given an exclusive legislative mandate to superintend the health care of the nation, allopathic medical practices were more uniform. A clearer appreciation by patients that, in today's world, uncertainty over the treatment of breast cancer can lead one specialist to recommend surgery and others to recommend radiation treatment or chemotherapy—all of which may be viable alternatives—could in itself moderate the evils of specialization.

Great tensions are created by the conflict between the quest for certainty and the reality of uncertainty. The resolution of these tensions in favor of certainty has been abetted by a number of assumptions of what constitutes good patient care. I now want to explore some of the assumptions that emphasize the importance of faith, hope, and reassurance, rather than of ambiguity and doubts, in the treatment of disease.

The Placebo Effect of the Physician

The importance that physicians have attributed throughout medical history to faith, hope and reassurance seems to demand that doctors be bearers of certainty and good news. Therefore, the idea of acknowledging to patients the limitations of medical knowledge and of doctors' capacities to relieve suffering is opposed by an ancient tradition. The controversy over the employment of placebos, whose effectiveness supposedly depends so much on the certainty with which they are prescribed by doctors and accepted by patients, provides a specific example of the tensions between faith and certainty, on the one hand, and acknowledgment of uncertainty, on the other. Therefore, an examination of the function of placebos in the contemporary practice of medicine—since their employment can be viewed as an attempt to hide lack of knowledge and uncertainty—may contribute to setting limits on the need for certainty in physician-patient interactions.

Traditionally placebos have been defined as any pills, potions or procedures whose effectiveness is not attributable to their pharmacologic or specific properties.[31] This definition only scratches the surface. Let me postpone looking more deeply into the definition and ask a question first: Why has the use of placebos been defended so apologetically and embarrassedly by their advocates and been attacked so vehemently by their opponents? That their use constitutes deceptive practice cannot be the whole answer, for the need for deception in the practice of medicine has had many defenders. For example, the lack of full disclosure of postoperative risks is justified on the ground of speeding recovery. Nor can the answer be found in the nonscientific basis of placebo treatments, for doctors continue to employ therapeutic agents such as steroids, chemotherapy and antibiotics for many diseases, even though the scientific rationale for their use remains obscure. Recently, one of my students made the astute observation that the controversy over placebos brings to the surface more acutely and undeniably the discomfort physicians have generally experienced over the fact that the effectiveness of so many of their practices is strongly influenced by symbolic powers that reside in the silent laying on of hands and is not merely a result of their scientific treatments.[32] The demonstrable effectiveness of placebos affirms this reality and contradicts the prevailing idea that only biological agents and specific physical interventions are curative. Moreover, placebos point to the need to assign psychological influences emanating from doctors, and not only from patients, a respectful place in the cure of disease. Thus, the discomfort that placebos engender in the hearts and minds of physicians may have to do less with an uneasiness over dishonesty, full disclosure, or a lack of knowledge of their scientific rationale, and more with a disquiet over the implications of placebo treatments for the overall practice of medicine.

For example, if placebos were to be acknowledged as effective in their own right, it would expose large gaps in medicine's and doctor's knowledge about underlying mechanisms of cure and relief from suffering. Whatever embarrassment such admissions would create, acknowledgment of placebos' effectiveness would also demand their incorporation into the practice of medicine as significant adjuvants to good medical care. To keep such disturbing problems out of mind, physicians either have interdicted the employment of placebos altogether or have used them furtively or secretly. Placebos deserve a different fate. Physicians must ask: What is the inherent strength in placebos that makes them such a powerful ally to treatment? It cannot reside in the pill itself, for by definition it is an inert substance. The answer has to be found elsewhere. Let me begin with a brief bit of history to give further support to the power of placebos throughout the ages.

Commentators on placebo treatment generally agree with W. R. Houston's observation that "[t]he great lesson . . . of medical history is that the placebo has always been the norm of medical practice, that it was only occasionally and at great intervals that anything really serviceable, such as the cure of scurvy by fresh fruits, was introduced into medical practice."[33] Only during the last 150 years, with the advent of medical science, has it become possible to distinguish between the therapeutic effects of interventions based on their pharmacologic and other specific properties, on the one hand, and on "X-factors" (placebos), on the other. These X-factors have been variously defined as residing in the symbolic healing import of either the intervention or the physician-intervenor. Here a complicating factor enters: Cure may have nothing to do with the intervention or the intervenor, for it could be due to a third factor—*vis medicatrix naturae*, the healing power of nature, i.e., the human capacity for self-healing.

Even in today's world it is difficult to sort out the contributions that these three factors—the placebo, the treatment, and the healing power of nature—make to cure. In the treatment of many diseases—for example, diabetes, angina pectoris and malignant neoplasms—a significant placebo effect can operate. Its impact on cure was dramatically affirmed in a scientific study to test whether the relief of severe anginal pain was a result of the surgical ligation of the internal mammary arteries or a placebo effect.[34] The study demonstrated the equally significant relief of anginal pain from a mere skin incision under anesthesia. The patients who underwent that sham procedure had been led to believe that they were being subjected to a ligation of their internal mammary arteries, an operation that hitherto had been considered a specific treatment for such conditions.

Placebos often produce not only dramatic cures, but also the same side effects as active medications. In addition, they can alter laboratory values and other measures of objective physiologic change, such as electrocardiograms. Thus, Howard Brody correctly concluded, "it is impossible to use placebo response to distinguish between a real, organic symptom and a symptom that is 'all in the patient's head,' although the myth to the contrary still persists."[35]

Since the placebo effect cannot reside in the pill, potion or treatment, investigators have begun to look elsewhere. In his seminal article, *The Doctor Himself as a Therapeutic Agent*, Houston perceptively observed that, in bygone days, physicians were shrewd observers skilled in dealing with human emotions and that doctors' ministrations were effective "in direct proportion to the faith that the doctor had and the faith that he was able to inspire in his patients."[36] He concluded that "[physicians] themselves were the therapeutic agents by which cures were effected."

If physicians themselves are the placebos, then they are powerful therapeutic agents in their own right. Their effectiveness is probably augmented by the positive transferences patients bring to their interactions with physicians. It is also likely that the placebo effect is unconsciously mediated. Deep in patients' unconscious, physicians are viewed as miracle workers, patterned after the fantasied all-caring parents of infancy. Medicine, after all, was born in magic and religion, and the doctor-priest-magician-parent unity that persists in patients' unconscious cannot be broken. The placebo effect therefore attests to the power of the unconscious. Yet, patients are defined by their consciousness as well. On a conscious level, patients are aware of the limitations of medicine and physicians. They have learned of these limitations from personal suffering, from illnesses and deaths of loved ones. Patients know that miracles are only occasionally the lot of mankind. They may hope for miracles, but they are also resigned to the reality of their rarity.

Two interrelated questions can now be asked: Will acknowl-

edgment of the limitations of medicine and of physicians undermine the placebo effect? And will not expressions of hope and reassurance cement faith and augment the placebo effect? Let me
first comment on the second question. It can only be answered
affirmatively. The evidence of the positive impact of a doctor's
reassuring pronouncements on patients is overwhelming. Thus
when the placebo effect and the patients' self-healing capacities
work together and patients get well, one can only ask: Why not
accept this remarkable gift that human nature has bestowed on
us? But often patients do not improve. Then they can only feel
deeply disappointed and deceived. Are hope and reassurance
worth this price?

A new question arises: Can hope and reassurance be offered
to patients without resorting to deception and without inviting
disappointment? Or put in terms of my initial question: Must acknowledgment of the limitations of medicine and of physicians
undermine the placebo effect? Here the answer is not as clear.
Such acknowledgments may indeed reduce that initial sense of
well-being that magnificent promises engender. Yet, acknowledgment of limitations leaves plenty of room for hope and faith.
Patients do get well. The unconscious and transference here
come to the aid of physicians and patients. Both factors will exert
their influence if physicians can be trusted. Moreover, uncertainty itself comes to the aid of their interactions because it too
leaves room for hope and faith. Therefore it may turn out that an
acknowledgment of uncertainty will enhance physicians' therapeutic effectiveness, because it demonstrates honesty in the face
of uncertainty and a willingness to be more engaged with their
patients than is possible when communications are beset by evasions, half-truths, and even lies. Patients hear these things, even
if they dismiss them at first and bask in the heady transference
feelings that, as I have suggested in Chapter VI, are prominent
early in treatment. It must also be recognized that the failure to
acknowledge uncertainty can create a sense of psychological
abandonment in patients that is as real as physical abandonment, for the withholding of crucial information compromises
intimacy, and physicians and patients can only engage in arm's-
length transactions. If that happens, the placebo effect is undermined rather than strengthened.

If one surveys these unresolved questions, another one arises
that may point us in the right direction: What kinds of faith,

hope, and reassurance do patients wish to place in and obtain from a doctor? The answer may very well turn out to be that patients hope that physicians can be trusted to observe carefully, to treat them with care, to alleviate unnecessary suffering, to discuss with them the implications of uncertainty's inevitable presence, to give the unpredictable forces of nature a helping hand, and, above all, to remain honestly present and not abandon patients when they need them most.

Supposedly, it was the reassurance of nonabandonment provided by physicians in the horse-and-buggy days of medicine, when they had so little else to offer, that patients found so comforting. I am not sure whether physicians behaved in such a fashion then or whether this attribution to a bygone age confuses actual and personal history and thus expresses infantile memories of a mother-healer's nonabandoning presence when she alleviated suffering by attending to her infant with comforting hands and sounds. Whatever the historical truth, the promise of non-abandonment, of a caring and honest presence that can underlie faith, hope, and reassurance in the face of the limitations of medical knowledge, may be what patients seek to find in doctors as therapeutic agents, and not doctors' promise to do the impossible. Impossible promises—even when only made implicitly as they so often are—leave patients with a sense of distrust that is difficult to reverse.

If physicians were to provide hope and reassurance in a more honest fashion, then the placebo effect of doctors would augment faith in new ways, and the need to resort to placebo-pills and placebo-treatment would be markedly reduced, if not eliminated. Placebos no longer will have to be employed to hide uncertainty and ignorance. Instead, physicians and patients may gradually learn that the placebo effect is an integral and inevitable component of the practice of medicine, that it constitutes its art and augments its science.

Physicians need to learn how to utilize their inherent placebo effect so that their scientific treatments will achieve full effectiveness. To attain this objective, placebos must not be employed to satisfy patients' demand for treatment, to hide diagnostic or therapeutic ignorance, to save doctors' time, or to make money. Such deceptive practices have been correctly decried. Instead, the placebo effect of physicians must be incorporated into the scientific practice of medicine.

The revolutionary change in medical practice ushered in by the age of science can be summed up as follows: while before, treatment consisted almost entirely of the placebo effect, it is now *both* placebo effect and science. Seen in this light, the contribution of the placebo effect to the relief of suffering need no longer be an embarrassment. It can be frankly acknowledged and its employment studied and defined.

Placebo pills or potions per se may then be relegated to museum shelves, making them relics of the past, like the goat dung and ground "unicorn" horns so freely dispensed by ancient physicians. Doctors alone will become the placebos, and they may not have to resort to spurious hope, faith, and reassurance to exercise their powerful effect. Such false premises may only undermine doctors' placebo effect and, in turn, disclosure and consent.

Finally it must be recognized that traditional justifications for placebos, faith, hope and reassurance have served physicians' needs to disregard uncertainty and profess certainty instead. Their use perpetuates the silence that has haunted doctor-patient interactions throughout history. It inhibits questioning of recommendations by and with physicians. Placebo pills, unrealistic faith, hope, and reassurance are powerful conversation stoppers. Thus, their administration serves doctors' interests in silent compliance in order to avoid the embarrassment of having to reveal so much about the uncertainties of medicine to lay persons and the problems of discussing such difficult matters with patients. Doctors are concerned about whether they have been equal to the task of explaining their recommendations to patients, particularly whenever patients decide not to follow their advice altogether or opt for a "less-preferred" alternative. These problems should not be taken lightly. They do not necessarily speak, however, to the intrinsic incomprehensibility of medicine's uncertainties; they address instead the willingness of doctors to learn how to talk with their patients about medicine's uncertainties.

Intervention or Delay

If the lack of candor about uncertainty cannot be justified solely by patients' needs, one must look elsewhere. Perhaps a closer look at some other problems inherent in the practice of medicine may shed light on the pervasive disregard of acknowledging uncertainty. I shall focus here on medicine's considerable ignorance about the respective contributions that *vis medicatrix naturae*—the healing power of nature—and doctor's interventions make to the healing process. These uncertainties in medical knowledge raise a most vexing question: When is nonintervention just as salutary as intervention? Traditionally, doctors have resolved this question by resorting to action on the assumption that doing something is better than doing nothing and out of a belief that errors of commission are less reprehensible than errors of omission.[37] Acting on such assumptions and beliefs also relieves the tension of living with the harmful consequences of any delay in the face of uncertainty, particularly since harm caused by mistakes of intervention can readily be ascribed to the natural progression of the underlying disease process. While delay is beset by uncertainty, too, errors of omission can more easily be blamed on physicians than can errors of commission. Acknowledgment of uncertainty about intervention or delay to patients would compel both to share responsibility for the decision ultimately made.

Physicians have also justified their tendency to intervene on the ground that patients demand that something be done for them. Doctors have overlooked, however, the contributions of their own long-standing preference for resolving any ambiguity about treatment in favor of intervention to the creation of such "demands." Fostering such expectations in patients makes acknowledgment of uncertainty about action or delay unnecessary, since both parties seemingly share the same preference. Yet, the preference for treatment over watchful waiting has many consequences. It can make patients out of persons who do not need to be so confirmed and who should be educated to rely more on their own self-healing capacities. It exposes such patients unnecessarily to the iatrogenic complications of the powerful treatments of modern medical technology, when either no treatment or a less drastic therapy is a viable alternative.

In a posthumously published paper, Franz J. Ingelfinger, the editor of *The New England Journal of Medicine*, noted the high incidence of patients' visits to doctors for illnesses that are either self-limited or beyond the curative capabilities of medicine.[38] He quoted the frequently given high figure of 90 per cent, but since "substantiating data [were] fragmentary," he did not state whether he believed the figure to be actually that high. His observations attest to the importance of an unexplored phenomenon. They also attest to the need for physicians not only to become more aware of their ignorance about when to delay and when to intervene, but also to acknowledge these uncertainties to patients. The high rate of "unnecessary" surgery, of resort to antibiotics and to tranquilizers, bears testimony to physicians' propensity to resolve uncertainty and ambiguity by action rather than inaction. To turn the tide requires a massive reeducation of physicians and patients. Both must learn that there is considerable value in living with uncertainty and not resolving it preemptorily in favor of action. The latter course imposes its own risks to life and health and its own considerable economic costs to individuals and society. Lest I am misunderstood, let me note that I favor neither action nor delay, but only the proposition that both are meaningful alternatives and that ultimately a patient must decide which route to follow. The traditional certainty with which intervention has been defended has obscured the uncertainties which beset such recommendations.

The Conflict between Art and Science

A related problem resides in the uncertainty of whether to base the practice of medicine on its modern science, its ancient art, or both. Even though the age of science has been with us for over one hundred years, the commitment to its scientific principles, appearances notwithstanding, is not solidly established within the medical profession. A telling example is the recent rush to coronary bypass surgery, a costly and hazardous procedure, based largely on clinical judgments rather than carefully controlled and reasonably conclusive experimental studies.[39] Nor have many older procedures, like tonsillectomies and hysterectomies, been subjected to rigorous verification despite considerable doubts about whether such interventions are indicated as frequently as they are being performed.[40] The uncertainties tend to be resolved by appeals to clinical judgment—the practice of the art of medicine—even though medicine's science, which is a better judge of the merits of the procedure than is clinical experience, cannot confirm such judgments. At a minimum, the conflicts between medicine's art and science should be brought to patients' awareness.

Professional Authoritarianism and the Mask of Infallibility

The lack of acknowledgment of uncertainty to patients is also reinforced by the traditional authoritarian relationship that governs interactions between physicians and patients and that doctors seek to foster. Professing certainty serves purposes of maintaining professional power and control over the medical decision-making process as well as of maintaining an aura of infallibility. Physicians' power and control are maintained not only by projecting a greater sense of certainty than is warranted but also by leaving patients in a state of uncertainty, not in the sense of shared uncertainties but in the sense of keeping patients in the dark. In a review article that is critical of such practices, H. Waitzkin and J. D. Stoeckle have persuasively argued that:

> *[A] physician's ability to preserve his own power over the patient in the doctor-patient relationship depends largely on his ability to control the patient's uncertainty.* The physician enhances his power to the extent that he can maintain the patient's uncertainty about the course of illness, efficacy of therapy or specific future actions of the physician himself.
>
> *   *   *
>
> . . . The less uncertain the patient becomes about the nature of his illness and the effects of treatment, the less willing he may be to relinquish decision-making power to the physician. . . .[41]

Doctors' acknowledgment of their uncertainties would significantly lessen this source of patient manipulation.

Donning a "mask of infallibility" is another way of maintaining professional control. Samuel Gorovitz and Alasdair MacIntyre observed that "[a]t present the typical patient is systematically encouraged to believe that *his* physician will not make a mistake, even though what the physician does may not achieve the desired medical objectives and even though it cannot be denied that some physicians do make mistakes."[42] They went on to point out that

[t]he first reaction of physicians to the invitation to dispense with the mask of infallibility is likely to be a humane alarm at the insecurity that a frank acceptance of medical fallibility might engender in the patient. But we wonder whether the present situation, in which the expectations of patients are so very often disappointed during medical treatment, is not a greater source of insecurity.

Physicians would admit to each other in private that infallibility eludes them, but they would at the same time also assert that they often have to conduct themselves vis-à-vis patients as if they possessed it. Masks can deceive not only the audience but the actor as well. The mask of infallibility makes it more difficult than it otherwise would be for physicians to explore their own doubts and uncertainties, and precludes acknowledging them to patients. Moreover, since infallibility is cousin to omnipotence, patients often are unwittingly led to expect too much from doctors' interventions and later will bitterly complain about the result obtained. Physicians then generally overlook the fact that such "ungrateful patients" are their own creation.

Acknowledgment of fallibility could bring uncertainties into the open and reduce the possibility of a misunderstanding based on mixed messages in doctors' orders, which occur whenever doubts remain unexpressed. More generally, it could reduce the existing gulf of inequality between physicians and patients and make its own contribution to a better appreciation that both are voyagers on the high sea of uncertainty. The extent to which patients can and wish to interact with doctors on such an unaccustomed basis, as I have suggested in Chapter VI, is unclear. At a minimum, however, some patients do wish to be treated in this manner. It will only become apparent how many patients feel this way once the curtain of silence, of mistrust in patients' capacities to engage in conversation, is lifted.

The Fear of Quacks and Concern over Costs

Two additional arguments that physicians have advanced against the acknowledgment of uncertainty deserve consideration. One speaks to fears that such revelations will drive patients into the arms of quacks who promise so much more, and the other speaks to concerns about the economic costs of more thorough-going conversations between physicians and patients. With respect to the first argument, I do not wish to suggest that a shift in professional practices toward greater acknowledgment of uncertainty will satisfy all patients or indeed, that it will not penalize some patients for whom blind faith in physicians is therapeutic. There are persons—but we do not know how many or how few—who wish to be confirmed as patients, who wish to escape from the painful and overwhelming vicissitudes of their lives by viewing themselves as incapacitated by physical illness. There are others who have an inordinate need for reassurance that everything can and will be set right. There are still others whose profound credulity makes them search for miracle workers and who will be bitterly disappointed if they cannot find them in their physicians. William Osler understood this well:

> The history of medicine is full of instances of self-deception on the part of the best of men, and it is well that the young man should be humble, as he is not likely to escape altogether. Science has done much in revolutionizing mankind, but man remains the same credulous creature as he has been in all ages. Tar-water, Perkin's tractors, laying on of hands, Christian Science, Lourdes, and other miracle-working shrines illustrate the deep, intense credulity from which science has not yet freed mankind and is not likely to do so. It is an aspect of human nature which we must accept and sometimes utilize, remembering the remark of Galen: "He cures the greatest number in whom most men have most faith."[43]

Doctors have insufficiently sorted out when patients' expectations of miracles should be challenged and when not, and, above all, what problems a submission to such expectations poses for physicians and the practice of scientific medicine.

Perhaps those patients who need miracle workers do not belong in doctors' offices. Yet physicians have all too unquestioningly accepted the burden of being healers to all the ills of mankind. This self-imposed duty, based in part on the highest motives of not turning suffering persons away, is also in need of reexamination. The commonly advanced justifications that patients have nowhere else to turn or that they must be kept away from nonphysician healers who will only endanger their health by administering quack remedies are unsatisfactory.

If, after doctors have acknowledged their limitations and promised only that they will try to do their best, patients decide to turn to faith healers, so be it. Physicians should not foreclose such moves by patients, if only to reassure the vast majority of patients who remain in their care that physicians will exercise only those skills they truly possess. Acting out of fear that any acknowledgment of medicine's limitations will drive patients into the arms of quacks has its own dangers. In promising more than medicine can deliver, physicians adopt the practices of quacks and are themselves transformed into quacks.

With respect to the economic argument, let me first observe that, particularly in recent years, physicians have been accused along with quacks of being guided more by economic than therapeutic considerations in the conduct of their practices. It has been asserted, for example, that the performance of radical surgery for breast cancer over less extensive procedures is influenced too much by the higher fees that the former operation commands, that appropriate referrals to other medical specialists are impeded by prospects of losing a fee, and that organized medicine's fight against nonmedical practitioners, including quacks, is dictated largely by economic considerations. While there is truth in these contentions, too much has been made of them; other less obvious but equally important issues that affect therapeutic practices adversely have been overlooked. I have been chided, and correctly so, that in my prior writings I have made too little of these economic pressures. At the same time, I still hold to the view that doctors' unwillingness to come to terms with their uncertainties about what properly falls within the domain of scientific medicine—whether to base their evaluation of a patient's condition on scientific or intuitive grounds, whether to delay or to intervene, and whether or not to share with patients their bafflement and even ignorance—influence their propensity to err on the side of intervention as much as do economic considerations. In not facing up to all these issues, doctors and patients have become victims of too many unnecessary interventions. That there is money to be made out of all this is true, but it is not the whole story.

Physicians themselves have employed economic arguments by contending that greater fidelity to disclosure and consent will be costly both in physicians' time and patients' fees. While the concern over cost must be taken seriously, it is not at all clear how much time conversation will take once doctors know what needs to be talked about, and how and why they should talk.

Moreover, physicians have always maintained that cost should not be an impediment to good patient care. If conversation with patients constitutes good patient care, then the expense can be justified on this ground. Physicians have not been averse to justifying the high costs of renal dialysis and coronary bypass surgery on the grounds that they are essential to good patient care. Furthermore, conversations about medical uncertainty may in fact reduce costs, for patients may decline interventions once they learn that they are optional rather than medically necessary. Once these and other issues have been scrutinized it may turn out that physicians' concerns over the economic costs of conversation may also mask an underlying concern: avoidance of the uncomfortable role of being the bearer of uncertainty.

I have tried to identify the formidable obstacles that the disregard of uncertainty poses for meaningful conversation between physicians and patients. I also have tried to suggest, that, despite the vast ignorance and uncertainty indigenous to the contemporary practice of medicine, it is not ignorance and uncertainty per se that constitute the problem, but the fear of and resistance to acknowledging uncertainty. If disclosure and consent are ever to have meaning, physicians must learn to manage uncertainty better than they have in the past.

Coping with Uncertainty

The question of how to moderate the defensive disregard of uncertainty must now be addressed. Not surprisingly, the poet, John Keats, points the way. As Freud frequently observed, writers and poets are possessed of remarkable psychological insights from which we can profit. Shortly before Christmas of 1817, Keats wrote to his brothers about a "disquisition" he had had with his friend Charles Wentworth Dilke, a very intelligent but highly doctrinaire young man:

> I had not a dispute but a disquisition with Dilke on various subjects; several things dove-tailed in my mind, and at once it struck me what quality went to form a Man of Achievement, especially in Literature, and which Shakespeare possessed so enormously—I mean *Negative Capability*, that is, when a man is capable of being in uncertainties, mysteries, doubts, without any irritable reaching after fact and reason. . . .[44]

He went on to say that "if pursued through volumes, [it] would perhaps take us no further than this, that with a great poet the sense of Beauty overcomes every other consideration, or rather obliterates all consideration."

In an essay on Keats' letters, Lionel Trilling observed that Keats tried to convey that in obliterating "all considerations of what is disagreeable or painful," one betrays the sense of Beauty, resulting in "a statement that really has no meaning."[45] Trilling juxtaposed Keat's letter to his brothers with his famous poem "Ode on a Grecian Urn" and its closing lines

> 'Beauty is truth, truth beauty,'—that is all Ye Know on earth, and all ye need to know.[46]

Trilling went on to observe, that like Shakespeare and other great poets, Keats looked at human life not only in terms of beauty but also in terms of its "ugly or painful truth."[47] Thus, unlike Dilke, whom Keats described as "a man who cannot feel that he has a personal identity unless he has made up his mind about everything," Keats emphasized the capacity for negative capability, "the faculty of not having to make up one's mind about everything." Trilling commented that this capacity depends "upon the sense of one's personal identity and is the sign of personal identity. Only the self that is certain of its existence, of its identity, can do without the armor of systematic certainties. To remain content with half-knowledge is to remain with contradictory knowledges; it is to believe that 'sorrow is wisdom' and also that 'wisdom is folly.'"

Keats knew illness; he had not walked the hospital wards for nothing. He was concerned with the "truth which is to be discovered between the contradiction of love and death, between the sense of personal identity and the certainty of pain and extinction." Physicians need to be like poets and in two senses. They are practitioners of the art of medicine, an art akin to that of the poets, who seek to discover beauty in its life affirming and life destroying dimensions. Yet, they are also practitioners of the science of medicine who seek to discover truth in the beauty of discovery and in the ugliness of ignorance.

Thus, physicians need to be educated not only to "a more reasonable awareness of uncertainty, a less dogmatic clinging to presumed certainties, a greater ability to face uncertainty with equanimity,"[48] as John C. Whitehorn has put it, but also to learning how to remain "in uncertainties, mysteries, doubts, without any irritable reaching after fact and reason."[49] What has been neglected in professional training is learning how truly to cope with uncertainties, how to avoid paying mere lip service to them and becoming paralyzed by them.

What I suggest here expands on my discussion in Chapter VI of the need for a greater awareness of countertransference. The quest for certainty and the denial of uncertainty I believe, must also be viewed as professional and personal countertransference problems. To come to terms with uncertainty is neither easy nor fully realizable, but it can be better taken into account than it has been.

It is possible to escape the tyranny of first impressions and naive preconceptions. Consider once again Halsted's radical mastectomy or coronary bypass surgery or the implantation of pacemakers. A greater appreciation of inevitable medical uncertainty could have led to more modest initial claims of the effectiveness of these procedures and to their less aggressive employment until effectiveness had been more clearly established. The example of penicillin, so frequently cited as a warning against delay, is not apposite. Its effectiveness was quickly established for a great many conditions that had been beyond medical control before its discovery. That its administration also had other consequences, discovered only later, like allergic sensitivity reactions or resistance to effectiveness, only speaks to what is true for all medical interventions: They must be administered judiciously.

If greater awareness and acknowledgment of uncertainty are too much to ask, at least it must be recognized that, in physician-patient interactions, professionals' defenses against ignorance and uncertainty are a greater problem than patients' ignorance. Such recognition will shift the burden of improving their conversations from patients to doctors. Moreover, shifting the focus from the uncertainty of medical knowledge to the ways in which professionals have coped with these uncertainties again places the burden on medicine's practitioners.

Patients' supposed intolerance of medical uncertainties may thus turn out to be a reflection less of an inherent incapacity to live with this tragic fact and more of an identification with the perceived incapacity of physicians to live with it. Patients' supposed intolerance may turn out to be significantly affected by a projection of physicians' intolerance onto patients. If so, then new paths can open up for trust. It could now travel along a two way street, from patient to doctor and from doctor to patient. Trust could be grounded in a mutual recognition of the capacities and incapacities of both parties for coping with human (professional and patient) vulnerabilities engendered by uncertainty.

Every physician is at the core also a patient, and every patient a healer. An admonition inscribed on a Greek temple spoke to this fact over two thousand years ago: "These are the duties of a physician: first . . . to heal his mind and to give assistance to himself before giving it to anyone (else). . . . Therefore he would not . . . increase his pretensions . . . but art . . . heart."[50] Art, heart, and science require new duties of physicians: to heal their minds of pretensions, to confront first within themselves and then with their patients, *their own* personal and professional uncertainties; and above all to trust conversation and to trust their patients as much as they themselves wish and expect to be trusted. Then Marcel Proust's observation that "in the light of medical error recognized only after years' time, to believe in medicine [is] the height of folly," would not loom as ominous as it has.[51] Instead, his accompanying observation would be even more apt than in days past: "not to believe in medicine [is] the greater folly still, for from this mass of errors there have emerged in the course of time many truths."

Summing up

The practice of medicine is beset by great uncertainty. Indeed, advances in medical knowledge notwithstanding, for a long time to come, if not forever, its practice will be accompanied by considerable ignorance. It is the legacy of science that scientific activity produces not only new knowledge but also new ignorance. There is a bright side, however. Since doctors are now better situated than they ever have been to make distinctions between the known, the unknown, and the unknowable, they can be better aware of, and converse more knowledgeably with patients about, medicine's uncertainties. Thus, uncertainty and ignorance of knowledge are not inimical to shared decision making between physicians and patients.

The disregard of uncertainty defeats the sharing of the burdens of decision. Its disregard has made a significant contribution to the duplicities, evasions, and lies that have infiltrated conversations with patients and made meaningful disclosure and consent a charade. Patients rightfully have felt cheated; whether they will feel equally cheated by an acknowledgment of uncertainty remains to be seen.

A better appreciation and, in turn, a better management of uncertainty will not emerge out of more refined technical medical knowledge, but rather out of the physician's and patient's psyches where, after all, certainty and uncertainty are perceived, judged, evaluated, and prepared for expression. The attempt to moderate the defenses against the disregard of uncertainty is worth the effort for a number of reasons: (1) it would lighten physicians' burdens by absolving them from the responsibility for implicitly having promised more than they or medicine can deliver; (2) it would give patients a greater voice in decision-making; (3) it would greatly reduce the exploitation of unwarranted certainty for purposes of control rather than care; and (4) it would significantly reduce the feelings of psychological abandonment that patients experience whenever they sense that doctors are withdrawing behind a curtain of silence or evasion. In the final chapter of this book, I would like to explore the feelings of abandonment that physicians' silence engenders in patients.

VIII

The Abandonment of Patients: A
Final Argument Against Silence

THE HISTORY OF MEDICINE is the history of physicians' caring but silent devotion to what they believed their patients' best interests dictated. Doctors were rarely heard to invite patients to share the burdens of decision with them. Instead, the voices heard were those of doctors' hopeful and reassuring promises, however truthfully, evasively or deceptively made, of doctors' orders, however gently or harshly uttered, and of patients' compliant assent, however cheerfully or resentfully given. The odd lack of conversation about physicians' hopes, doubts, and expectations and about patients' wishes, fears, and expectations—odd once one begins to contemplate how little they talked with one another about matters of crucial importance to both—made patients feel abandoned and confused. When physicians did not listen to patients, or responded perfunctorily to their questions, or dismissed their doubts and concerns, patients felt abandoned. While patients' childlike wishes and needs to be relieved of all responsibility for their care were well attended to, their adult wishes and needs to be informed, heard, and consulted were utterly disregarded. As a result, they felt confused about their simultaneous but contradictory feelings of being cherished and abandoned.

The focus of this chapter is on the abandonment that patients experience as a result of doctors' reluctance to involve them in the process of thinking about choices and of making final decisions jointly. Beyond all the arguments for and against shared decision making explored in this book—authority, self-determination, psychological autonomy, and uncertainty—the most significant argument in its favor resides in the fact that doctors' distrust of patients' decision-making capacity constitutes an abandonment of patients. In this concluding chapter I shall first describe the sense of abandonment that patients experience in their interactions with physicians, and then explore how doctors' fears of death and assumptions about patients' similar fears foster a lack of communication that undermines mutual decision making. The fear of death hovers over all physician-patient encounters and not only over those with dying patients.

The core of the argument in what follows is this: Ultimately disclosure and consent seek to pierce the isolation, to eliminate the feelings of abandonment, and to reverse the lack of control that patients now experience so often in their interactions with physicians. Put affirmatively, disclosure and consent seek to safeguard patients' integrity that, illness notwithstanding, doctors can either help restore or undermine further; or put another way, disclosure and consent seek to protect patients from the ravages and pain of abandonment. Thus, the idea of informed consent is grounded not only in the principle of self-determination but in good therapeutic management as well, for relief of suffering requires doctor's presence in the full sense of the word. What is therapeutic for citizens turns out to be equally therapeutic for patients. Perhaps the ancient debate to the contrary can now finally be laid to rest.

Psychological Abandonment

By abandonment I do not mean physical abandonment which physicians have always considered one of the gravest violations of their ethical commitment to good patient care, but rather, psychological abandonment. Physicians have overlooked that, even while physically present, they tend to become estranged from their patients because of their attitudes toward and interactions with them. The estrangement between physicians and patients that evokes increasing feelings of abandonment in patients has one of its roots in the self-estrangement that illness mobilizes. When ill, patients experience themselves as not fully in control of their bodies and minds. Suddenly, they are more in touch with unaccustomed feelings of fright, dependence, neediness, precariousness, and insecurity—feelings that they generally either have kept under control or have disregarded, except in instances of identifiable external danger.

Patients bring this sense of self-estrangement to doctors' offices on their first visit. In addition, they bring to their appointment other feelings that have not been given the attention they deserve. Even before their initial meeting, patients have formed an intense bond with the doctor, engendered by a positive transference-readiness that is rooted in infancy, re-evoked by illness, and fed by hopeful expectations that the doctor will not only relieve their physical suffering but also assist them in being more fully in charge of themselves once again. While patients come to the appointment as if an intense relationship with their physician has already been forged, doctors do not have to accept this unilateral psychological "contract." Indeed, they should not until other matters have been clarified. They must appreciate that if they merely accept patients' "contract," without first exploring patients' ill-sorted out expectations of what doctors will and can do for them, disappointment and resentment over unfulfilled "promises" may eventually haunt their relationship.

Soon after physicians and patients meet, the latters' feelings of personal estrangement are reinforced rather than relieved, by doctors' perception and treatment of patients as they exchange the status of person for that of patient. In viewing patients too much as needy children, physicians disregard the fact that patients are adults as well. In seeing only the neediness engendered by suffering and fear, physicians overlook other of their patients' needs: to know what ails them, what can make them better, and what their prospects are. Patients may wish to know all these things so that they can take better charge of their life during illness as they have been accustomed to being in charge of their life during health.

Doctors' ready retreat behind silence—apparent to patients by doctors' demeanor when they keep most of their thoughts to themselves, deprive patients of vital information, or pat patients on the back and assure them that everything will be all right and that they need not worry—makes patients feel disregarded, ignored, patronized, and dismissed.

Since, from patients' vantage point, a relationship between them and their doctor exists, they begin to feel psychologically abandoned as individuals. They experience themselves as having become merged with the featureless mass of all their doctor's patients. Initially, patients are only dimly aware of such reactions because their incipient feelings of abandonment are obscured by wishes to surrender to and merge with a powerful healer. But, as time goes on, particularly when illness does not readily respond to treatment, feelings of psychological abandonment mount and are more acutely experienced. They are as tormenting as feelings of physical abandonment, perhaps even more tormenting, because physical abandonment can more easily be identified and responded to by patients, while the source of psychological abandonment is much harder to identify and deal with. Patients may wonder whether their feelings of abandonment are of their own making, a response to their own "insatiable" neediness and greediness. They may then react to nagging feelings of guilt that such views of themselves can engender by asking even fewer questions or by trying to suppress conscious resentment toward their doctor over their aloneness. Regardless of whom patients blame, their feelings of abandonment persist, increase in intensity, and cause confusion because the source of such feelings remains unclear.

Patients' feelings of abandonment can confuse them in other ways as well. Since they are gratified by doctors' attentiveness to their childlike wishes of caretaking, patients may view themselves as ungrateful when they become aware of feelings of resentment over not being treated "properly." The confusion becomes augmented because patients only dimly recognize that by "properly" they mean that the doctor has treated them too much as the children they once were but no longer are. And patients are doubly confused because of their own complicity in the process, both by having experienced pleasure in being treated as children and by not having voiced their resentment about the assault on their dignity and self-respect.

The following story illustrates the impact on patients of such barely recognized feelings. Some time ago, a successful businessman who was widely admired for his philanthropy and involvement in civic affairs told me at a dinner party of his long bout with a mysterious illness which had taken him to many medical centers until it was finally diagnosed and successfully treated. He had no resentment about the failure to identify the cause of his illness earlier because he knew that he had suffered from a rare disease that was difficult to diagnose. Yet, as he talked about his experience, he became increasingly agitated and angry. Finally, he stopped himself and asked: "Why do I always get so angry when I tell this story? I should be, and indeed I am, grateful to all the physicians for having employed their skills to track down the cause of my obscure illness. They finally did and ever since then I have been free of pain and suffering. I am grateful and yet I also am not."

Since he had spoken of his medical Odyssey at length, I had learned many details about his interactions with his doctors. I said to him, "I think I know what makes you so angry. You are a person whom everybody treats with considerable respect. Yet, once you entered the hospital, everybody from young interns on up called you by your first name, while they expected you to address them as 'doctor.'" Of course, that aspect of their interactions was only one example of the disregard of his adult status, but it had affected him deeply. I had noticed how his anger mounted whenever he referred to the ways he and the doctors had addressed each other by name. After my comment, he spoke movingly about the difficulties he had experienced in conversing with his doctors on the basis of mutual respect; they had made him feel so childlike. At the end of the evening, he sought me out again and told me that he now could place the episode in better perspective. He felt even more grateful for his doctors' dedication to his physical welfare and for their technical skills, but now he also knew that the next time he would ask to be called Mr. _____ or request permission to address his doctors by their first names. He appreciated that this was only an opening move, but a consequential one, toward a more respectful interaction between himself and his doctors.

Many patients intuitively feel that good caretakers should not permit them to surrender passively, and they are correct. Doctors are under an obligation to invite their patients to think with them, to work collaboratively toward a decision. Since illness is a situation of neediness and fear, it stimulates wishes to surrender to authority and fantasies about omnipotent caretakers to whom one must yield. These wishes and fantasies should not be exploited by physicians, even though at first such an exploitation seems to make doctors' interactions with compliant patients easier. Since the deprivation of information magnifies fears of the unknown, physicians' silence intensifies such wishes and fantasies. Conversation, on the other hand, might strike a better balance between patients' ambivalent wishes of being taking care of and of taking care.

At bottom, patients resent physicians' lack of trust of their capacities to participate in the decisions that are so crucial, so personally important, to patients' future well-being. Physicians have been puzzled by patients' resentment, particularly in this century, when they have much to offer their patients. Yet, patients' resentment would begin to make sense if the abandonment they experience, not of their bodies but of their persons, were more clearly recognized.

Thus, it is not only illness and anxiety over illness that account for the dehumanizing estrangement and, in turn, for the feelings of abandonment. Doctors contribute significantly to such feelings by the way they talk or do not talk, listen or do not listen. When doctors provide only bits and pieces of information, they further obscure the crucial matters that deserve mutual exploration: alternatives, delay, risks, benefits, uncertainties, quality of life, hopes, fears, doubts, and expectations. Without a sharing of such vital information, physicians and patients become estranged from one another; recommendations become orders and advice becomes command.

To be sure, when recovery from illness is uneventful and complete, patients tend to make little of these experiences. But when outcome or the treatment process itself, as is so often the case, does not agree with patients' fantasied or realistic expectations, they gradually become more aware of feelings of abandonment, although they may not identify them as such. Instead, they may complain that their doctor is too busy, is preoccupied with sicker patients, is disinterested in their complaints, or speaks a language they cannot understand. While no physician can ever be totally present, the point I wish to emphasize is that the iatrogenic deprivation of information makes a powerful contribution to patients' sense of abandonment.

The Exploitation of Death

I shall explore the general problem of silence and abandonment by using clinical material that largely is derived from physicians' interactions with dying patients. I do so for two reasons; the first is a practical one. The issue of abandonment has been identified and described best by observers and commentators in situations of impending death and thus they provide the richest source material for analysis. Using such examples runs the danger of obscuring the similarities and differences between abandonment in terminal and nonterminal situations. I would like to draw attention to that danger and to the need to study and analyze these differences. At the same time, I believe that the materials from physicians' interactions with dying patients only highlight the general problem of abandonment that affects all physician-patient relationships in which silence or withdrawal from respectful conversation and interaction is a significant factor.

A second reason for the relevance of such clinical material is that death has a special place in the practice of medicine. Since illness tends to mobilize thoughts of death, the presence of death as an invisible third party in doctors' offices distinguishes medicine from most other professions. Its dominion is magnified by physicians' reluctance to acknowledge its presence, either as a realistic concern or as an imaginary participant. To speak of death is difficult. Except when ill, most human beings prefer to deny death and the certainty of their mortality.

My experiences as a psychoanalyst, confirmed by many colleagues, have made me realize how rarely, even during a prolonged psychoanalysis, patients talk about their own death or reflect on the implications of their eventual death for the conduct of their time-limited existence in this world. Death, rather than sex or aggression—as has often been postulated—seems to be the most taboo subject. What is true for patients is equally true for physicians.

The silence that surrounds death, however, does not only reside in the discomfort that the topic engenders. Physicians' silence also serves the purpose of reinforcing their authority over patients. Doctors have an intriguing love-hate relationship with death: It is both their ally and their enemy. In trying to defeat death, physicians are death's adversaries. When physicians borrow the power engendered by patients' fear of death for purposes of control, death is their ally. Doctors often wittingly and unwittingly exploit the anxieties and fears that even benign illness engenders in patients by conveying, if not with words then by demeanor, that not following their orders will accelerate death. For example, take the following admonition contained in the first Code of the American Medical Association: "A patient who has . . . selected his physician, should always apply for advice in what may appear to him *trivial* cases, for the most *fatal* results often supervene on the *slightest* accidents."[1] Parsons also fell victim to physicians' exploitation of the fear of death for purposes of control when he wrote "[a]ll the physician can say to the patient who refuses to heed his advice is 'well, it's your own funeral'— which it may be literally."[2] Survival, however, is often not an issue. Yet fears of death are not dispelled since they serve well purposes of control, obedience, and compliance.

Physicians' aversion to talk about death imperceptibly blends with their wishes to control decision making. Both contribute to the failure to distinguish between situations where death may have to be acknowledged and the more usual situations where death's power can be assigned to a distant and uncertain future. The reluctance to talk about death when it is an issue has come to include situations in which talking about death would only lay to rest patients' unwarranted concerns about dying.

Strange as it may sound, physicians' struggle against and embrace of death can cast a dark shadow over another covert struggle between physicians and patients: how life is to be lived. Life, including the life of illness, can be lived in myriads of ways, and not only according to the views of physicians. Yet, doctors allow the spectre of death to hang ominously over many treatment recommendations—such as a recommendation for the surgical removal of a uterus because fibroid tumors *might* turn into cancer, or for the removal of a gallbladder because silent gallstones could act up at a time when a patient *might* be physically incapacitated to tolerate the stresses of surgery well—and without clearly and insistently specifying the remoteness of such deathly outcomes. Such exploitation of death reinforces doctors' control and impairs patients' capacity to make their own decisions. It serves physicians' interests more than those of patients.

Interactions with Dying Patients

I now turn to related considerations in interactions with dying patients. As I have observed, death is physicians' adversary and friend. It is also dying patients' adversary and friend, but for different reasons. For dying patients, death means separation from the living but it may also mean relief from the inevitable process of dying. These differing views of physicians and patients about the adversarial and friendly nature of death need to be kept in mind. Otherwise, for example, doctors may fight death too vigorously as an adversary, while for dying patients it may be an ally promising welcome deliverance, not so much from pain but from suffering. Eric Cassell has persuasively argued that pain and suffering must be distinguished. In a poignant article, he observed that "it is not uncommon for suffering to occur not only during the course of a disease but also as a result of its treatment."[3] He also made the point that "the obligation of physicians to relieve human suffering stretches back into antiquity [but] little attention is explicitly given to the problem of suffering in medical education, research, or practice."

A better appreciation of suffering can teach us that extension of life is one, but not the only, objective of medicine. Thus, how to think about remaining life and come to terms with it needs to be separated from how to think about dying and come to terms with it. Physicians who do not talk about the life of terminal illness and how various treatments will affect it, and who readily assume that patients share their views on longevity, overlook the suffering they cause patients by taking away the choices that illness still leaves open to them. That, too, constitutes an abandonment.

The reluctance to talk about death with the dying out of concern for their welfare must also be evaluated against evidence that seems to suggest that the dying have less of a problem talking about their impending death than do other living persons.[4] Thus, greater responsibility for the "conspiracy of silence" in these contexts may have to be assigned to physicians alone, and not to physicians and dying patients. If this view is correct, we once again encounter the phenomenon of projection—in this case, the attribution of physicians' beliefs to dying patients. Such projections are reinforced by physicians' general reluctance to talk with patients about matters that could lead to a sharing of the burdens of decision.

Before I continue, I should emphasize that there are no substantial data that document a detrimental impact on patients of disclosure of dire prognoses.[5] While physicians are apt to refer to stories of severe depression or suicide following such disclosures, documentation of such evidence is difficult to obtain. Veatch has reported that "[a] director of a major suicide prevention center has said that there is no evidence of an abnormally high suicide rate after revelation of cancer or other terminal diagnosis."[6] Veatch added that he has "been able to find no such evidence." In this connection, Edwin Shneidman, who has studied the phenomenon of suicide, made the cogent observation that the question that deserves study is "why so many cancer patients *do not* commit suicide."[7] Nor have many in-depth studies been conducted of how patients react subsequent to the initial disclosure of dire prognosis. Suggestive evidence indicates that patients handle such news in a variety of ways, including denial, passive acceptance, and active acceptance (e.g., by living life intensely, volunteering for medical experiments, or seeking recourse to other healers, including faith healers). On the other hand, these facts should not be taken to imply that satisfactory evidence exists in support of the beneficial impact on patients of revelations of dire prognosis. At best, one can only point to our collective ignorance about an important problem.

Despite the absence of solid data on both sides, the prevailing belief among physicians still seems to be that patients should not be fully informed about dire prognoses, that expressions of hope and reassurance are preferrable to a realistic appraisal of patients' conditions. I believe this to be a correct assessment of the current climate of medical opinion even though more patients are being informed of their diagnosis than was the case in the past. But what has happened is that the physicians' silence has shifted from diagnosis to the treatment process. In earlier years, physician's treatment options were limited. Today, thanks to the advances in medical science, a great many therapeutic modalities are available and, in order to employ them, doctors have been forced to make some statement about diagnosis. To the extent patients are better apprised about diagnosis, they are not adequately informed about the risks and benefits of treatment alternatives, including those of no treatment. Instead, in the service of aborting meaningful conversation, doctors liberally dispense hope and reassurance to obfuscate patients' understanding of their chances of benefiting from treatment. Thus, patients continue to remain deprived of opportunities to make their own decisions. As a consequence they feel isolated, alone, and abandoned, even though they may try hard to deny such feelings by clinging to the hopeful reassurances that their physicians provide.

It is certainly correct to assume that some dying patients wish to know their real condition so that they can remain in charge of their ebbing life, and that others prefer to be deceived. But we have not learned how to distinguish those patients who prefer to know from those who prefer to be deceived. We cannot distinguish between them as long as physicians continue to treat most patients as if they did not wish to know more about what lies ahead. Identifying patients who wish to know more about their prospects invites their participation of how to proceed in the light of such revelations. Physicians, however, have little experience in engaging in conversations with any patients—be they terminally ill or not—that could lead to shared decision making. The problem of how to interact with the dying is only a specific example of a more general problem. Thus, in learning not to abandon dying patients, physicians may also learn not to abandon patients in general.

The Denial of Death

Interactions between physicians and dying patients will not improve substantially until doctors have a better appreciation of their own reactions to talking with patients about death, and consequently being constantly reminded of their own mortality. Physicians must learn to manage these reactions better if they wish to carry out their professional responsibilities toward patients. This is not an easy assignment for, as I have already suggested, an awareness of death may be a greater problem for those whose prospects of dying are remote than it is for those who are terminally ill. Freud asserted that "at bottom no one believes in his own death, or, to put the same thing in another way, that in the unconscious every one of us is convinced of his immortality."[8] In his book, *The Denial of Death*, Ernest Becker expressed the need for denial in more desperate words, "the idea of death, the fear of it, haunts the human animal like nothing else; it is a mainspring of human activity—activity largely to avoid the fatality of death, to overcome it by denying in some way that it is the final destiny for man."[9] William Jones said it sardonically: "[let] sanguine healthy-mindedness do its best with its strange power of living in the moment and ignoring and forgetting, still the evil background is really there to be thought of, and the skull will grin in at the banquet."[10]

After reviewing these and other statements, Becker was led to the conclusion that "a full apprehension of man's condition would drive him insane" because "[m]an is literally split in two, he has an awareness of his own splendid uniqueness in that he sticks out of nature with a towering majesty, and yet he goes back into the ground a few feet in order blindly and dumbly to rot and disappear forever. It is a terrifying dilemma to be in and to have to live with."[11]

Freud came to different conclusions. He believed that human beings can face up to their mortality. He noted that the "civilized attitude toward death," based on a variety of psychological and religious defenses and convictions, suggests that "we are once again living psychologically beyond our means."[12] He asked, "Should we not rather turn back and recognize the truth? Would it not be better to give death the place in reality and in our thoughts which is its due, and to give a little more prominence to the unconscious attitude towards death which we have hitherto so carefully repressed?" He then proceeded to answer his own question:

> . . . This hardly seems an advance to higher achievement, but rather in some respects a backward step—a regression; but it has the advantage of taking the truth more into account, and of making life more tolerable for us once again. To tolerate life remains, after all, the first duty of all living beings. Illusion becomes valueless if it makes this harder for us.
>
> We recall the old saying: *Si vis pacem, para bellum.* If you want to preserve peace, arm for war.
>
> It would be in keeping with the times to alter it: *Si vis vitam, para mortem.* If you want to endure life, prepare yourself for death.

Yet as Becker observed, Freud's is a lonely voice. Thus it is not surprising that, because of their own psychological needs, physicians have preferred reassuring and hopeful nondisclosure to disclosure of reality in situations of impending death. In pointing to the unfortunate consequences for patients that supposedly follow revelations of dire prognosis, doctors have neglected to identify their own fears and anxieties that such conversations engender.

Fears of death seem to be unusually prominent among physicians. In a study conducted by Herman Feifel and his colleagues, a group of 81 physicians was compared with a group of seriously ill and terminally ill patients and with another group of 95 healthy individuals.[13] The physicians were significantly more afraid of death than were the healthy or the dying lay persons. When Feifel and his associates also compared a group of medical students with experienced physicians, they found that the latter were more fearful of death than the former. This finding suggests that contact with death increases physicians' fears. Feifel's results have been corroborated by other researchers.[14] These studies provide strong evidence that the avoidance to talk about death and dying is reinforced by the fears that such conversations evoke in physicians. Moreover, doctors view death as a personal defeat rather than an eventual inevitability to which they, like their patients, must submit. As long as death is viewed as a failure, it is difficult to talk about it. One does not like to speak of one's failings.

Arguments against Disclosure of Dire Prognosis

The traditional arguments against disclosure of dire prognosis have largely been based on two concerns: that such revelations may cause sudden death, and that they create needless suffering for the remainder of patients' lives. I shall take up each in turn.

The existence of a causal relationship between strong emotions, particularly fear, and sudden death has been supported by anecdotal examples since the beginning of recorded history. St. Luke's report that Ananias was struck dead on the spot immediately after Peter said to him, "You have not lied to man but to God,"[15] has been attributed by secular physicians to overwhelming fright. In more recent times, Walter Cannon's classic article, "Voodoo Death," has been widely quoted in support of the notion that emotions can cause sudden death.[16] One of the most

compelling of Cannon's stories dates back to 1692. It was first reported by a traveller to the Congo who had not witnessed the
event himself but had repeatedly been told about a healthy young
African who had died shortly after having been informed that
some years earlier a friend had surreptitiously fed him a break-
fast of wild hen. Eating such food was strictly banned by his
tribal rules. Other more contemporary cases of Voodoo death
have made much of the deadly impact of curses on persons whose
belief systems seem to make them vulnerable to such incanta-
tions.[17]

While today such religious and magical beliefs do not seem to
affect Western man as they perhaps once did, their rare though
powerful influence should not be discounted. The belief that serious illness, particularly cancer, is divine punishment for all kinds
of misdeeds has not been completely laid to rest in Western culture. There have been scattered reports of patients turning their
faces to the wall, becoming listless, and dying within days, after
being informed that they suffered from fatal illnesses.[18] These
deaths could very well have been due to deep-seated beliefs that
God was finally punishing these patients for misdeeds and sins
they had committed in fantasy or reality. Such cases document
the power of forces, be they religious, magical, or biological, beyond human control. Since they are very rare events, such deaths
should not lead one to the sweeping generalization that nondisclosures of dire prognosis make sense for all patients.

Moreover, these reports are flawed by the fact that sudden
death particularly from cardiovascular causes is not a rare phenomenon. The incidence of sudden deaths ranges from 10–32
percent of all deaths due to natural causes.[19] Thus, even when
disclosures of prognosis have been made, it is not clear whether
death was the result of physiological or emotional causes. Many
examples of Voodoo deaths, including Cannon's, are flawed because emotions may only have caused death indirectly. Instead,
it may have been due to physiological causes such as starvation
and dehydration, for often the victims refused food and water out
of a belief that they had been bewitched and that death was inevitable.[20] This could have been the fate of one of my patients.

During a tour of duty as a medical officer in the Air Force, a
young airman born in Puerto Rico was admitted to my ward because of his "refusal" to eat. He was visibly wasting away and
death from starvation seemed imminent. He told me that he
wanted to eat but could not. He sadly remarked that eating

would not make any difference anyway because his mother-in-law in Brooklyn had fashioned a doll in his image into which she had inserted straws in order to suck out his vital fluids. She was angry with him for having married her daughter. I tried, but to no avail, to discuss with him the irrationality of his beliefs. Even several attempts at forced feeding did not reverse his downhill course. With each succeeding day he became weaker. Fortunately, when I realized that my powers were insufficient to counteract those of his mother-in-law, it occurred to me to ask whether anyone else could help.

His face brightened, and he told me of a conjurer in Mississippi who would be able to remove the hex that his mother-in-law had placed on his life. I immediately called him, explained the situation, and asked for his help. A letter addressed to the airman arrived in time. My Mississippi colleague explained what he had done in his office to counteract the mother-in-law's activities. He assured our patient that he would soon be well. Indeed, our patient quickly recovered and returned to active duty. Thirty years later, I am still awed by this event to which I contributed only a willingness to interact with my patient on his own terms, to bow to his belief system when mine seemed powerless against his, to trust his convictions, and to consult with others more adept at treatment of such diseases than I was or ever could be.

I do not intend to enlist these examples to prove that strong emotions either can or cannot be implicated as a cause of death. I only wish to highlight the paucity of data, the frequent references to cultures removed from ours, and the existence of alternative explanations for the phenomenon of sudden death. In the light of these considerations, it is most questionable to draw any conclusive inferences about the inadvisability of disclosure of dire prognosis. Moreover, since acting on such data interferes with patient choice, the contrary data—for example, that awareness of prognosis, combined with a psychological determination to fight for survival, improves life expectancy for those patients who are so predisposed—deserve particular attention, if only to emphasize once again our ignorance.

This brings me to the second concern: that revelation of dire prognosis causes patients needless suffering. This contention must also be examined against the background of the suffering engendered by non-disclosure of such an undeniable truth. In their comprehensive article on "Predilection to Death," Avery Weisman and Thomas Hackett stressed the dangers of non-disclosure: "Tacitly to impose silence, denial, deception, and isolation upon the dying patient may itself cause suffering and bring about bereavement of the dying, a state of premortem loneliness, emotional abandonment, and withdrawn interest."[21] Many of their examples testified to the fact that "patients would be willing to discuss death, if the doctor were only able to overcome his own guilt or anxiety enough to permit it." One of their cases supports their thesis most poignantly. A doctor who had convinced himself that his patient was not aware of his fatal condition had avoided talking about many things with his patient, including the doctor's own grief over his patient's imminent death. Finally the doctor's sentiments got the better of him and on a last visit he

> was moved to pity by the futility of his patient's plight. It was obvious that life could not continue and that there was little to say except good-bye. As the doctor sat silently, he sadly put his hand on the patient's shoulder. The patient glanced at him and wrote on a pad of paper: "Don't take it so hard, doc!"

This encounter, representative of many others, illustrates the deathly estrangement-in-life between physician and patient which silence or spurious reassurance and hope engender.

Weisman and Hackett also emphasized that a lack of candor about prognosis strips patients of all control over the life still ahead of them, cruelly abandoning them instead to a world of silence that soon enough will be their fate. Modern technology has gone too far in providing life supports that attach patients only to caretaking bottles and not to caring hands, that speak in voices of caretaking monitors but not of caring tongues. I do not wish to romanticize dying, as some have done. That, too, constitutes a dangerous evasion. I only wish to suggest that the pain of dying can be made worse by silence, that we may have been wrong in believing that maintaining spurious hope is usually preferrable. Dylan Thomas offered one alternative by asserting that anger over dying need not be avoided:

> Do not go gentle into that good night.
> Rage, rage against the dying of the light.[22]*

*Dylan Thomas, *Poems of Dylan Thomas*. Copyright 1952 by Dylan Thomas. By permission of New Directions Publishing Corporation. Dylan Thomas, *Collected Poems*. Published by J. M. Dent. By permission of David Higham Associates Limited.

The pain of anger can perhaps be tolerated better than the pain of premature abandonment.

Weisman and Hackett also suggested that the process of dying, particularly the suffering from premortem loneliness, is more fearsome to patients than death itself. The silent isolation that the healthy impose on the dying by furtive and evasive contacts can only augment such fears. Therefore, conversation-stopping hope and reassurance are not the answer.

Hope and reassurance need to become an echo, a creative act of reflecting back to patients what physicians can truly promise after they know more about their patients, their illnesses and their expectations, rather than an uniformed opening move that discourages conversation. How physicians can spare patients unnecessary pain and suffering, and how they should treat or not treat patients depend ultimately on patients' individual needs and expectations, factors that only conversation can reveal. But such conversations can only become meaningful if physicians are prepared to seize every opportunity their patients provide for talking more truthfully about their medical prospects and about what they, as their doctors, can do for them. A willingness to do so will create a climate of trust between physicians and patients that now does not exist.

To be sure, the evidence as to how many patients wish to talk about their impending death, and indeed would welcome such an opportunity still needs to be gathered. A most personal experience illustrates our ignorance about patients' wishes. Years ago, a distinguished surgeon operated on my mother. On finding a cancer that had spread widely from its original site, he appropriately decided to do nothing. Prior to the exploratory operation, he had frequently visited my mother, and both had enjoyed talking with one another. After the operation he rarely made an appearance and, when he did, he left hastily. My mother became upset by what she took to be a sign of disrespect. Moreover, she experienced his conduct as an abandonment, as an important loss, because she had enjoyed so much her conversations with this bright, intelligent, and witty person. She wondered what she had done to offend him and asked me to find out what had happened.

When I spoke with him, he told me first of his anguish over having failed her, particularly since in his preoperative encounters with my mother he had been so reassuring about her eventual recovery. He also was at a loss as to how to deal with questions of what was wrong with her and of her impending death. For these reasons, he had made himself so scarce. When I reassured him that it was most unlikely that she would raise such questions unless he invited them, he returned to her bedside. She felt "honored" by his visits and they gave her much pleasure during her remaining weeks. She never expressed any conscious awareness of her dying, though I believe she knew more than she divulged. I shall never know whether she remained silent out of a belief that it would spare her three sons additional pain or whether she did not want to learn the truth. I did not help her to decide for herself; indeed, I probably gave her all kinds of signals not to talk about her impending death. She died at a time when my prior socialization as a physician, which had taught me not to talk about death, had too unquestioned a hold on me.

In being too reassuring and hopeful in his initial encounters with her, my mother's surgeon felt trapped and at a loss to remain engaged with her after he had discovered that the malignancy was beyond control. This consequence is not the only painful price to be paid for not taking greater care with words that promise too much. Already in the initial encounters with patients, the undiscriminating expression of hope and reassurance creates doubts in patients and their families about whether doctors can be trusted. Countless anecdotal examples attest to patients' deep-seated beliefs that all reassurance may be just a ploy to hide the truth about the patient's dire condition, even—and this is a tragic consequence frequently overlooked—when it is a true assessment of a patient's favorable prognosis. What Richard C. Cabot said about lying to patients—that a lie cannot be isolated like "a case of smallpox," but that it spreads "far beyond our intention and our control," and that it "[begets], as a rule, . . . a quiet, chronic incredulity which is stubborn"[23]—also holds true for indiscriminate hope and reassurance. They, too, become suspect, even when truthfully given.

The need to learn how to administer hope and reassurance more caringly and carefully becomes even more apparent if one examines other misuses such practices have invited. Obliterating the certainties and uncertainties inherent in any conversation about dire prognosis by resorting to euphemisms such as "we'll never know for sure," or withholding information about the gravity of patients' conditions can only confuse patients, since the rosy picture the doctor is projecting does not agree with their own intuitive evaluation of their condition. It can leave patients with a nagging sense of doubting their own judgment, if not their sanity.

One dying woman expressed this well, in demeanor and words, when her doctor finally told her that she was not "nervous" but dying: "The smile she gave [her doctor] actually expressed relief. 'Thank God,' she said, 'Someone's finally told me the truth.' "[24] The truth about her impending death, however painful, liberated her from isolation; from the madness of doubting her own sanity; from the abandonment that she experienced as she listened to her doctors, nurses, and family, all of whom talked largely about trivialities and not about real concerns; and from the abandonment created by furtive contacts to avoid revealing the truth inadvertently.

There is much here that requires intensive study. It may then turn out, as I believe it will, that physicians' reluctance to share the burdens of decision making with the dying does not reflect doctors' special concerns about this group of patients but is only another manifestation of their general tendency to exclude patients from such participation. If I am correct, then shared decision making would at the end of patients' lives pierce the silence that has haunted them throughout their lives as patients.

If it turns out that the abandonment dying patients experience as a result of the silence that separates them from their physicians is only a dramatic illustration of the abandonment experienced by all patients, then shared decision making is more than a right to which patients are entitled; it becomes a therapeutic necessity because it alleviates unnecessary suffering. Therefore, if we are willing to listen to the dying, they can leave us a rich legacy that will only accrue to the benefit of future generations of patients, whether terminally ill or not.

Summing up

Throughout this book I have observed that faith, hope, and reassurance have too often served physicians' needs to maintain authoritarian control, to hide uncertainties, and to facilitate patients' regression to more infantile modes of functioning in order to encourage nonverbal interactions and compliance. If some physicians seek to justify such conduct on grounds of medical necessity and their benign and altruistic intentions, they must also recognize the fateful consequences of their demands for compliance: the surrender of autonomy and independence, with all that such surrender implies about patients' inevitable disappointment over physicians' inability to deliver on the promise of total caretaking and, in turn, about the inevitable feelings of abandonment that such disappointment mobilizes. If these consequences are considered unfortunate and in need of correction through conversation, then disclosure and consent are vindicated not only by libertarian values of safeguarding citizens' freedom to pursue their own destiny in their own self-willed ways but also by Hippocratic values of caringly attending to patients' needs.

I appreciate that I have given caring a new dimension, but in doing so I have only identified some long-neglected problems that have compromised physicians' commitment to caring and healing. Since ancient times, doctors have asserted that they are healers of all the medical ills of mankind. And medical ills, which physicians tend to define broadly, can encompass almost all aspects of living. While there is arrogance in such a vision, it need not remain arrogant. The vision can also be pursued with humility by tempering aspiration with an awareness and acknowledgment of the limits of both medical knowledge and the province of medicine. In individual interactions with patients, the arrogance that a vision of healer readily engenders can perhaps only be contained if doctors were to recognize that such a vision does not confer on doctors the right to make crucial decisions, without permission, for another person even if that person is a patient.

The resort to coercion, however subtly handled, has stalked the interactions between physicians and patients, as it has the interactions between human beings in general. If doctors could learn, and in turn teach their patients, that it is possible to sit down and reason together about the most important personal anxieties and fears that illness and its treatment engenders, then they could also point the way to living life not by submission but by mutual respect, with careful attentiveness to one's own and the other's rationalities and irrationalities. Living the life of medicine in such new and unaccustomed ways could extend the dominion of reason and thus make doctors true healers to mankind. In the absence of such a commitment doctors only perpetuate and reinforce the alienation between man and man. The root meaning of doctor is "teacher" (from the Latin *docere*, to teach or to instruct), and the root meaning of physician is "a natural philosopher" (from the Greek *physicos*, an inquirer into nature). The two meanings must be joined so that physician-doctors can fulfill their dual functions as inquirers into the ills of mankind and patients, and as Socratic teachers who seek to arrive at a truth in concert with patients.

The physician-patient relationship that I envision will not be easy to implement. Authoritarianism is deeply imbedded in professional practices. Fears about the awareness and acknowledgment of uncertainty loom large in physicians' and patients' psyches and the retreat from honest conversation is a powerful social reality. These forces that conspire against disclosure and consent cannot be taken lightly. They speak to the fact that the idea of informed consent does not now govern the relationship between physicians and patients, that its time has not yet come.

Before informed consent can become a viable principle, fundamental obstacles to its implementation must first be identified and removed. In this book I have tried to identify many of these obstacles and to suggest how they might be overcome. I have not tried to specify in any detailed fashion how physicians and patients must and can converse with one another. Instead, I have tried to identify the preconditions for informed consent and to draw attention to the consequences of its rejection.

In conclusion I would like to make a few brief observations on some of the objections to patient participation in decision making that surely will be raised. I have not spoken about conversing with "stupid" patients (or by whatever other more gentle euphemism such patients are called). I do not wish to deny their existence, although I wonder whether their number is as great as physicians commonly believe and whether the stupefying environment in which doctors and patients now live does not significantly increase their number. At a minimum, I would assert that a significant number of patients have the intellectual capacities for searching conversation and that they must be given a greater role in decision making.

Nor have I said much about the cost in physicians' time and patients' expense that conversation would entail. The railroading of patients, seeing scores of them a day back to back, surely would be affected by conversation. If physician income were to suffer as a consequence, then doctors' contemporary claims to a right to financial compensation, that has placed them near the top in earnings compared with other groups, must be reconciled with medicine's ancient claims to placing patient care first. At a minimum, those instances must be identified when conversation is crucial, that is, when it can be justified, irrespective of economic costs, because choices are complex, hazardous and irreversible in their consequences, and because alternatives, delay or doing nothing are viable options.

Moreover, informed consent could play a vital role in containing the much lamented explosion in medical cost. A greater clarity about the elective nature of many treatments—about the benefits of their employment or delay, and about the risks of intervention or delay—may change patterns of utilization of medical services in significant ways. The time costs of conversation may turn out to be much less than the costs of intervention. Of all proposals to contain the explosion in medical costs one has not received the attention it deserves: having patients play a more vital role in deciding whether to undergo tests and treatments that need not necessarily be performed. "Second medical opinions" may be one answer, but "first patient opinions" may be a better answer.

I said more, although still not enough, about the prevalent assertion that patients generally do not wish to share the burdens of decision and that they prefer instead to trust their doctors' recommendations blindly. I doubt this assertion. We shall not know whether I am right or wrong, however, until doctors are willing to make a good faith effort to invite patients' participation. This would obligate physicians to reassure patients that they will take the time to talk with them, that patients' doubts and questions will be given a respectful hearing, and that they are prepared to provide patients with sufficient information so that patients can formulate their questions in a meaningful fashion. Only when patients appreciate that the invitation is more than a gesture can doctors begin to make distinctions between patients' decisional preferences.

The radically different climate of physician-patient decision making that I envision cannot be implemented by judicial, legislative, or administrative orders. At best, such outside interventions can prod doctors; at worst, they only substitute bureaucratic authority for professional authority. Meaningful change can come about only through medical education and the education of patients. *Both* physicians and patients must rethink basic assumptions about their relationship and about mutual decision making. Physicians here must take the initiative and lead the way. Time will tell whether physician-educators will rise to this challenge not merely by paying lip service to the need for more "humanitarian" training in this age of medical technology but by a thorough and long overdue scrutiny of ancient professional beliefs about the proper treatment of patients and their diseases.

This task will not be pursued with the necessary seriousness, however, until we discard the dangerous notion that the complexities of physician-patient interactions can be resolved solely by trust in physicians' integrity, their compassion, and their commitment to the Golden Rule. The complexities inherent in the practice of medicine, in the conflicting motivations that physicians bring to their interactions with patients, and in the conflicting needs that patients bring to their interactions with physicians defy such appealing but simplistic notions. Instead, the problems that I have identified need intensive study and analysis. Of the many recommendations that will come forth from such explorations, one will most certainly be that physicians and patients must talk more with one another. And, in the context of such conversations, doctors' integrity and compassion, and even the Golden Rule, will make essential but not exclusive contributions to good patient care. One question will surely arise during these explorations: Can patients be trusted to participate more fully in the decisions that affect their well-being? The answer one gives to this question will shape the subsequent analysis of all the other problems. I believe that patients can be trusted. If anyone were to contest that belief, I would ask: Can physicians be trusted to make decisions for patients? This book has argued that both must be trusted, but that they can only be trusted if they first learn to trust each other.

APPENDIX A

Code of Ethics of the American Medical Association (1847)

CHAPTER I

OF THE DUTIES OF PHYSICIANS TO THEIR PATIENTS AND
OF THE OBLIGATIONS OF PATIENTS TO
THEIR PHYSICIANS

ART. I.—DUTIES OF PHYSICIANS TO THEIR PATIENTS

1. A physician should not only be ever ready to obey the calls of the sick, but his mind ought also to be imbued with the greatness of his mission, and the responsibility he habitually incurs in its discharge. Those obligations are the more deep and enduring, because there is no tribunal other than his own conscience to adjudge penalties for carelessness or neglect. Physicians should, therefore, minister to the sick with due impressions of the importance of their office; reflecting that the ease, the health, and the lives of those committed to their charge, depend on their skill, attention and fidelity. They should study, also, in their deportment, so to unite tenderness with firmness, and condescen-

Adopted by the American Medical Association May 1847. (All Articles that do not pertain directly to the physician-patient relationship have been deleted.)

230

sion with authority, as to inspire the minds of their patients with gratitude, respect and confidence.

2. Every case committed to the charge of a physician should be
treated with attention, steadiness, and humanity. Reasonable indul-
gence should be granted to the mental imbecility and caprices of the
sick. Secrecy and delicacy, when required by peculiar circumstances,
should be strictly observed; and the familiar and confidential intercourse to which physicians are admitted in their professional visits,
should be used with discretion, and with the most scrupulous regard to
fidelity and honor. . . .

3. Frequent visits to the sick are in general requisite, since they
enable the physician to arrive at a more perfect knowledge of the disease,—to meet promptly every change which may occur, and also tend
to preserve the confidence of the patient. But unnecessary visits are to
be avoided, as they give useless anxiety to the patient, tend to diminish
the authority of the physician, and render him liable to be suspected of
interested motives.

4. A physician should not be forward to make gloomy prognostications, because they savor of empiricism, by magnifying the importance of his services in the treatment or cure of the disease. But he
should not fail, on proper occasions, to give to the friends of the patient
timely notice of danger when it really occurs; and even to the patient
himself, if absolutely necessary. This office, however, is so peculiarly
alarming when executed by him, that it ought to be declined whenever
it can be assigned to any other person of sufficient judgment and delicacy. For, the physician should be the minister of hope and comfort to
the sick; that, by such cordials to the drooping spirit, he may smooth
the bed of death, revive expiring life, and counteract the depressing influence of those maladies which often disturb the tranquility of the most
resigned in their last moments. The life of a sick person can be shortened not only by the acts, but also by the words or the manner of a physician. It is, therefore, a sacred duty to guard himself carefully in this
respect, and to avoid all things which have a tendency to discourage the
patient and to depress his spirits.

5. A physician ought not to abandon a patient because the case is
deemed incurable; for his attendance may continue to be highly useful
to the patient, and comforting to the relatives around him, even in the
last period of a fatal malady, by alleviating pain and other symptoms,
and by soothing mental anguish. . . .

ART. II.—OBLIGATIONS OF PATIENTS TO THEIR PHYSICIANS

1. The members of the medical profession, upon whom is en-
joined the performance of so many important and arduous duties

towards the community, and who are required to make so many sacrifices of comfort, ease, and health, for the welfare of those who avail
themselves of their services, certainly have a right to expect and require, that their patients should entertain a just sense of the duties
which they owe to their medical attendants.

2.   The first duty of a patient is, to select as his medical adviser
one who has received a regular professional education. In no trade or
occupation, do mankind rely on the skill of an untaught artist; and in
medicine, confessedly the most difficult and intricate of the sciences,
the world ought not to suppose that knowledge is intuitive.

3.   Patients should prefer a physician whose habits of life are regular, and who is not devoted to company, pleasure, or to any pursuit in-
compatible with his professional obligations. A patient should, also,
confide the care of himself and family, as much as possible, to one physician, for a medical man who has become acquainted with the pecu-
liarities of constitution, habits, and predispositions, of those he attends,
is more likely to be successful in his treatment, than one who does not
possess that knowledge.

A patient who has thus selected his physician, should always apply
for advice in what may appear to him trivial cases, for the most fatal
results often supervene on the slightest accidents. It is of still more importance that he should apply for assistance in the forming stage of vio-
lent diseases; it is to a neglect of this precept that medicine owes much
of the uncertainty and imperfection with which it has been reproached.

4.   Patients should faithfully and unreservedly communicate to
their physician the supposed cause of their disease. This is the more important, as many diseases of a mental origin simulate those depending
on external causes, and yet are only to be cured by ministering to the
mind diseased. . . .

5.   A patient should never weary his physician with a tedious detail of events or matters not appertaining to his disease. Even as relates
to his actual symptoms, he will convey much more real information by
giving clear answers to interrogatories, than by the most minute account of his own framing. Neither should he obtrude upon his physician the details of his business nor the history of his family concerns.

6.   The obedience of a patient to the prescriptions of his physician
should be prompt and implicit. He should never permit his own crude
opinions as to their fitness, to influence his attention to them. A failure
in one particular may render an otherwise judicious treatment dangerous, and even fatal. This remark is equally applicable to diet, drink,
and exercise. As patients become convalescent, they are very apt to
suppose that the rule prescribed for them may be disregarded, and the
consequence, but too often, is a relapse. Patients should never allow
themselves to be persuaded to take any medicine whatever, that may
be recommended to them by the self-constituted doctors and doc-

tresses, who are so frequently met with, and who pretend to possess infallible remedies for the cure of every disease. However simple some of their prescriptions may appear to be, it often happens that they are productive of much mischief, and in all cases they are injurious, by contravening the plan of treatment adopted by the physician.

7. A patient should, if possible, avoid even the friendly visits of a physician who is not attending him—and when he does receive them, he should never converse on the subject of his disease, as an observation may be made, without any intention of interference, which may destroy his confidence in the course he is pursuing, and induce him to neglect the directions prescribed to him. A patient should never send for a consulting physician without the express consent of his medical attendant. It is of great importance that physicians should act in concert; for although their modes of treatment may be attended with equal success when employed singly, yet conjointly they are very likely to be productive of disastrous results.

8. When a patient wishes to dismiss his physician, justice and common courtesy require that he should declare his reasons for so doing.

9. Patients should always, when practicable, send for their physician in the morning, before his usual hour of going out; for, by being early aware of the visits he has to pay during the day, the physician is able to apportion his time in such a manner as to prevent an interference of engagements. Patients should also avoid calling on their medical adviser unnecessarily during the hours devoted to meals or sleep. They should always be in readiness to receive the visits of their physician, as the detention of a few minutes is often of serious inconvenience to him.

10. A patient should, after his recovery, entertain a just and enduring sense of the value of the services rendered him by his physician; for these are of such a character, that no mere pecuniary acknowledgement can repay or cancel them.

CHAPTER II

OF THE DUTIES OF PHYSICIANS TO EACH OTHER, AND TO THE PROFESSION AT LARGE

ART. IV.—OF THE DUTIES OF PHYSICIANS IN REGARD TO CONSULTATIONS

2. In consultations, no rivalship or jealousy should be indulged; candour, probity, and all due respect should be exercised towards the physician having charge of the case.

3. In consultations, the attending physician should be the first to propose the necessary questions to the sick; after which the consulting physician should have the opportunity to make such further inquiries of the patient as may be necessary to satisfy him of the true character of the case. Both physicians should then retire to a private place for deliberation; and the one first in attendance should communicate the directions agreed upon to the patient or his friends, as well as any opinions which it may be thought proper to express. But no statements or discussion of it should take place before the patient or his friends, except in the presence of all the faculty attending, and by their common consent; and no opinions or prognostications should be delivered, which are not the result of previous deliberation and concurrence.

*   *   *

6. In consultations, theoretical discussions should be avoided, as occasioning perplexity and loss of time. For there may be much diversity of opinion concerning speculative points, with perfect agreement in those modes of practice which are founded, not on hypothesis, but on experience and observation.

7. All discussions in consultation should be held as secret and confidential. Neither by words nor manner should any of the parties to a consultation assert or insinuate, that any part of the treatment pursued did not receive his assent. The responsibility must be equally divided between the medical attendants,—they must equally share the credit of success as well as the blame of failure.

8. Should an irreconcilable diversity of opinion occur when several physicians are called upon to consult together, the opinion of the majority should be considered as decisive; but if the numbers be equal on each side, then the decision should rest with the attending physician. It may, moreover, sometimes happen, that two physicians cannot agree in their view of the nature of a case, and the treatment to be pursued. This is a circumstance much to be deplored, and should always be avoided, if possible, by mutual concessions, as far as they can be justified by a conscientious regard for the dictates of judgment. But, in the event of its occurrence, a third physician should, if practicable, be called to act as umpire; and, if circumstances prevent the adoption of this course, it must be left to the patient to select the physician in whom he is most willing to confide. But, as every physician relies upon the rectitude of his judgment, he should, when left in the minority, politely and consistently retire from any further deliberation in the consultation, or participation in the management of the case.

ART. V.—DUTIES OF PHYSICIANS IN CASES OF INTERFERENCE

2.   A physician, in his intercourse with a patient under the care of another practitioner, should observe the strictest caution and reserve. No meddling inquiries should be made—no disingenuous hints given relative to the nature and treatment of his disorder; nor any course of conduct pursued that may directly or indirectly tend to diminish the trust reposed in the physician employed.

3.   The same circumspection and reserve should be observed when, from motives of business or friendship, a physician is prompted to visit an individual who is under the direction of another practitioner. Indeed, such visits should be avoided, except under peculiar circumstances; and when they are made, no particular inquiries should be instituted relative to the nature of the disease, or the remedies employed, but the topics of conversation should be as foreign to the case as circumstances will admit.

4.   A physician ought not to take charge of, or prescribe for a patient who has recently been under the care of another member of the faculty, in the same illness, except in cases of sudden emergency, or in consultation with the physician previously in attendance, or when the latter has relinquished the case, or been regularly notified that his services are no longer desired. Under such circumstances, no unjust and illiberal insinuations should be thrown out in relation to the conduct or practice previously pursued, which should be justified as far as candour, and regard for truth and probity will permit; for it often happens, that patients become dissatisfied when they do not experience immediate relief, and, as many diseases are naturally protracted, the want of success, in the first stage of treatment, affords no evidence of a lack of professional knowledge and skill.

CHAPTER III

OF THE DUTIES OF THE PROFESSION TO THE PUBLIC AND OF THE OBLIGATIONS OF THE PUBLIC TO THE PROFESSION

ART. II.—OBLIGATIONS OF THE PUBLIC TO PHYSICIANS

1.   The benefits accruing to the public, directly and indirectly, from the active and unwearied beneficence of the profession, are so numerous and important, that physicians are justly entitled to the utmost consideration and respect from the community. The public ought like-

wise to entertain a just appreciation of medical qualifications;—to make a proper discrimination between true science and the assumptions of ignorance and empiricism,—to afford every encouragement and facility for the acquisition of medical education,—and no longer to allow the statute books to exhibit the anomaly of exacting knowledge from physicians, under liability to heavy penalties, and of making them obnoxious to punishment for resorting to the only means of obtaining it.

APPENDIX B

American Medical Association Principles of Medical Ethics (1980)

The medical profession has long subscribed to a body of ethical statements developed primarily for the benefit of the patient. As a member of this profession, a physician must recognize responsibility not only to patients, but also to society, to other health professionals, and to self. The following Principles adopted by the American Medical Association are not laws, but standards of conduct which define the essentials of honorable behavior for the physician.

I. A physician shall be dedicated to providing competent medical service with compassion and respect for human dignity.

II. A physician shall deal honestly with patients and colleagues, and strive to expose those physicians deficient in character or competence, or who engage in fraud or deception.

III. A physician shall respect the law and also recognize a responsibility to seek changes in those requirements which are contrary to the best interests of the patient.

IV. A physician shall respect the rights of patients, of colleagues, and of other health professionals, and shall safeguard patient confidences within the constraints of the law.

Reprinted by permission of the American Medical Association, 1980.

V. A physician shall continue to study, apply and advance scientific knowledge, make relevant information available to patients, colleagues, and the public, obtain consultation, and use the talents of other health professionals when indicated.

VI. A physician shall, in the provision of appropriate patient care, except in emergencies, be free to choose whom to serve, with whom to associate, and the environment in which to provide medical services.

VII. A physician shall recognize a responsibility to participate in activities contributing to an improved community.

Notes

All unidentified citations in the text refer to the last preceding source marked in the Notes.

Introduction

1. Parsons, T., *The Social System* (New York: Free Press of Glencoe, 1951), p. 465.
2. See, for example, Davis, M., "Variations in Patients' Compliance with Doctors' Advice: An Empirical Analysis of Patterns of Communication," 58 *American Journal of Public Health* 274 (1968); Davis, M., "Variations in Patients' Compliance with Doctors' Orders: Medical Practice and Doctor-Patient Interaction," 2 *Psychiatry in Medicine* 31 (1971); Francis, V., Korsch, B., and Morris, M., "Gaps in Doctor-Patient Communication: Patients' Response to Medical Advice," 280 *New England Journal of Medicine* 535 (1969).
3. Solzhenitsyn, A., *Cancer Ward,* trans. N. Bethell and D. Burg. (New York: Bantam, 1969), p. 79.

4. Natanson v. Kline, 350 P. 2d 1093 (Kan. 1960).

5. Duff, R. and Hollingshead, A., *Sickness and Society* (New York: Harper and Row, 1968), p. 128.

6. Peabody, F., "The Care of the Patient," 88 *Journal of the American Medical Association* 877 (1927). Reprinted in 40 *Connecticut Medicine* 545 (1976).

7. Flexner, A., *Medical Education in the United States and Canada, Bulletin no. 4.* (New York: Carnegie Foundation for the Advancement of Teaching, 1910).

Chapter 1

1. 4 Hippocrates, *Aphorisms,* trans. W. Jones. (Cambridge: Harvard University Press, 1967), p. 99.

2. Natanson v. Kline, 350 P. 2d 1093 (Kan. 1960).

3. Canterbury v. Spence, 464 F. 2d 772 (D. C. Cir. 1972).

4. Natanson v. Kline, *supra* note 2, p. 1106.

5. *Oath of Hippocrates* (Fifth century B.C.).

6. 2 Hippocrates, *Decorum,* trans. W. Jones (Cambridge: Harvard University Press, 1967), p. 297.

7. Plato, 1 *Laws,* trans. R. Bury. (New York: Putnam's, 1926), p. 309 (Law 720).

8. Plato, *The Republic,* trans. B. Jowett. Book III, 3rd ed. (Oxford: Clarendon Press, 1888), p. 94.

9. *Ibid.*

10. Plato, 1 *Laws, supra* note 7.

11. *Ibid.*

12. In this and the next two paragraphs, I follow depictions of Greek medicine found in Entralgo, P., *Doctor and Patient,* trans. F. Partridge. (London: World University Library, 1969), pp. 45–51.

13. Plato, "Lysis." In: *The Collected Dialogues of Plato,* eds. E. Hamilton and H. Cairns (New York: Pantheon Books, 1961), p. 160.

14. 1 Hippocrates, *Precepts,* trans. W. Jones. (Cambridge: Harvard University Press, 1972), p. 319.

15. Plato, "Charmides." In: *The Collected Dialogues of Plato, supra* note 13, p. 103.

16. Entralgo, *supra* note 12, p. 186.

17. Entralgo, *supra* note 12, p. 209.

18. Welborn, M., "The Long Tradition: A Study in Fourteenth-Century Medical Deontology." In: *Medieval and Historiographical Essays in Honor of James Westfall Thompson,* ed. J. Cate and E. Anderson (Chicago: University of Chicago Press, 1938). Reprinted in *Legacies in Ethics and Medicine* (C. Burns ed.) (New York: Science History Publications, 1977).

19. The exact reference could not be located but Plato referred to physicians and the use of falsehoods in several of his writings. See, for example, Plato, "The Republic, Book III." In: *The Collected Dialogues of Plato, supra* note 13, line 389b.:

   But further we must surely prize truth most highly. For if we were right in what we were just saying and falsehood is in very deed useless to gods, but to men useful as a remedy or form of medicine, it is obvious that such a thing must be assigned to physicians, and laymen should have nothing to do with it.

   See also Plato, "The Republic, Book V," line 459d.

20. MacKinney, L., "Medical Ethics and Etiquette in the Early Middle Ages: The Persistence of Hippocratic Ideals," 26 *Bulletin of the History of Medicine 1* (1952). Reprinted in *Legacies in Ethics and Medicine, supra* note 18.

21. Hippocrates, *Decorum, supra* note 6, p. 289.

22. Margalith, D., "The Ideal Doctor as Depicted in Ancient Hebrew Writings," 12 *Journal of the History of Medicine and Allied Sciences* 37 (1957). Reprinted in *Legacies in Ethics and Medicine, supra* note 18.

23. Levey, M., "Medical Deontology in Ninth Century Islam." In: *Legacies in Ethics and Medicine, supra* note 18, pp. 136–37.

24. MacKinney, *supra* note 20.

25. Bar-Sela, A. and Hoff, H., "Isaac Israeli's Fifty Admonitions to the Physicians," 17 *Journal of the History of Medicine and Allied Sciences* 245 (1962). Reprinted in *Legacies in Ethics and Medicine, supra* note 18 (Admonition #31).

26. Welborn, *supra* note 18.

27. Bar-Sela and Hoff, *supra* note 25 (Admonition #38).

28. MacKinney, *supra* note 20.

29. 24 *Bulletin of the History of Medicine* 255 (1950). Reprinted in *Legacies in Ethics and Medicine, supra* note 18.

30. Gregory J., *Lectures on the Duties and Qualifications of a Physician* (Philadelphia: M. Carey & Son, 1817).

31. See, for example, Pernick, M., "The Patient's Role in Medical Decisionmaking: A Social History of Informed Consent in Medical Therapy." In 3 *Making Health Care Decisions* (President's Com-

mission for the Study of Ethical Problems in Medicine and Biomedical and Behavioral Research, 1982).

32. Rush, B. "The Progress of Medicine" and "The Vices and Virtues of Physicians" (1801). In: *The Selected Writings of Benjamin Rush*, ed. D. Runes (New York: Philosophical Library, 1947).

33. *Percival's Medical Ethics*, ed. C. Leake. (New York: Robert Krieger Publishing Company, 1975).

34. Percival T., *Medical Ethics* (Manchester 1803).

35. See, for example, Pernick, M., *supra* note 31.

36. Percival, *supra* note 33, p. 191.

37. Tolstoy, L., "The Death of Ivan Ilych." In: *Great Short Works of Leo Tolstoy*, trans. L. Maude and A. Maude (New York: Harper and Row, 1967), pp. 285–286.

38. Code of Ethics of the American Medical Association (adopted May, 1847), Chapter 1, Article I, Section 4.

39. Code of Ethics of the American Medical Association (adopted May, 1847), Preliminary Note.

40. Principles of Medical Ethics of the American Medical Association (adopted June, 1912), Chapter 2, Article III, Section 7.

41. Principles of Medical Ethics of the American Medical Association (adopted 1957), Section 1.

42. American Medical Association, Opinions and Reports of the Judicial Council (Chicago, 1957).

43. American Medical Association, Current Opinions of the Judicial Council (Chicago, 1981).

44. White, P., "Obituary-Richard Clarke Cabot," 220 *New England Journal of Medicine* 1049 (1939).

45. 5 *American Medicine* 344 (1903). Reprinted in *Ethics in Medicine: Historical Perspectives and Contemporary Concerns,* ed. S. Reiser, A. Dyck and W. Curran (Cambridge: Massachusetts Institute of Technology Press, 1977).

46. Ravitch, M., "The Myth of Informed Consent," *Surgical Rounds* 7 (February, 1978).

47. DeLee, S., "Malpractice and Informed Consent: A Legal Ploy," 61 *International Surgery* 331 (1976).

48. Laforet, E., "The Fiction of Informed Consent," 235 *Journal of the American Medical Association* 1579 (1976).

49. Coleman, L., "Terrified Consent," 11 *Physician's World* (May, 1974).

50. Ravitch, *supra* note 46.

51. Freud, S., "New Introductory Lectures on Psycho-Analysis." In: 17 *The Standard Edition of the Complete Psychological Works of Sigmund Freud* (London: The Hogarth Press, 1977).

52. MacIntyre, A., "Patients as Agents." In: *Philosophical Medical Ethics—Its Nature and Significance,* ed. S. Spicker and H. Englehardt (Boston: D. Reidel Publishing Company, 1977).

Chapter 2

1. In addition to the primary sources, this section on the history of the professions draws on the following:

Kett, J., *The Formation of the American Medical Profession: The Role of Institutions, 1780–1860* (New Haven: Yale University Press, 1968).

Carr-Saunders, A. and Wilson, P., *The Professions* (Oxford: Clarendon Press, 1933).

Brieger, G., ed., *Medical America in the Nineteenth Century: Readings from the Literature* (Baltimore: Johns Hopkins Press, 1972).

King, L., *The Road to Medical Enlightenment, 1650–1695* (New York: American Elsevier Publishing Company, 1970).

2. Starr, P., *The Social Transformation of American Medicine* (New York: Basic Books, 1982).

3. Kett, J. *The Formation of the American Medical Profession, supra* note 1, p. 5.

4. Bledstein, B., *The Culture of Professionalism: The Middle Class and the Development of Higher Education in America* (New York: Norton, 1976).

5. Massachusetts Colonial Laws (Boston, 1878), p. 28.

6. Bowman v. Woods, 1 Greene 441 (Iowa 1848).

7. Eastman v. State, 109 Ind. 278 (1887), quoting Hockett v. State, 105 Ind. 250 (55 Am. R. 201).

8. Thomson, S., *A Narrative of the Life and Medical Discoveries of Samuel Thomson . . . to which is added An Introduction to his New Guide to Health,* 2nd Ed. (Printed for the author by E. G. House, Boston, 1825), pp. 43–44.

9. Principles of Medical Ethics of the American Medical Association (adopted June, 1912), Chapter 2, Article I, Section 2.

10. Feinstein, A., "Clinical Biostatistics—XXVI. Medical Ethics and the Architecture of Clinical Research," 15 *Clinical Pharmacology and Therapeutics* 316 (1974).

11. Bledstein, B., *supra* note 4.

Chapter 3

1. Faretta v. California, 422 U.S. 806 (1975).
2. Slater v. Baker and Stapleton, 95 Eng. Rep. 860 (K.B. 1767).
3. State v. Housekeeper, 16 A. 382 (Md. 1889).
4. Pratt v. Davis, 118 Ill. App. 161 (1905).
5. Schloendorff v. New York Hospital, 211 N.Y. 125 (1914).
6. Pratt v. Davis, *supra* note 4.
7. Schloendorff, *supra* note 5.
8. Haskins v. Howard, 16 S.W. 2d 20 (Tenn. 1929).
9. Hunt v. Bradshaw, 88 S.E. 2d 762 (N. C. 1955).
10. See, for example, Canterbury v. Spence, 464 F. 2d 772, 784 (D.C. Cir. 1972); Cobbs v. Grant, 502 P. 2d 1 (Cal. 1972).
11. Shehee v. Aetna Casualty & Surety Co., 122 F. Supp. 1 (D.C. La. 1954).
12. Salgo v. Leland Stanford Jr. University Board of Trustees, 317 P. 2d 170 (Cal. Dist. Ct. App. 1957).
13. Katz, J., "Informed Consent—A Fairy Tale? Law's Vision," 39 *University of Pittsburgh Law Review* 137 (1977).
14. American College of Surgeons' Brief as Amicus Curiae in Support of Defendant and Appellant Frank Gerbode (1956).
15. Salgo, *supra* note 12.
16. Natanson v. Kline, 350 P. 2d 1093 (Kan. 1960).
17. See, for example, Carpenter v. Blake, 60 Barb. 488 (N.Y. Sup. Ct. 1871), reversed on other grounds, 50 N.Y. 696 (1872); Jackson v. Burnham, 20 Colo. 532; 39 Pac. 577 (1895), reversing 28 Pac. 250 (1891).
18. Fortner v. Koch, 272 Mich. 273, 261 N.W. 762 (1935).
19. Solzhenitsyn, A., *Cancer Ward*, trans. N. Bethell and D. Burg (New York: Bantam, 1969), p. 77.
20. Natanson, *supra* note 16.
21. Letter from attorney, dated August 28, 1978.
22. Natanson, *supra* note 16.
23. Harper, F. and James, F. Jr., *The Law of Torts* (Boston: Little, Brown & Company, 1956), Section 3.3, pp. 216–218.
24. Plante, M., "An Analysis of 'Informed Consent'," 36 *Fordham Law Review* 639 (1968).
25. Smith, H., "Therapeutic Privilege to Withhold Specific Diagnosis

from Patient Sick with Serious or Fatal Disease," 19 *Tennessee Law Review* 349 (1946).

26. Natanson, *supra* note 16.
27. Canterbury, *supra* note 10.
28. Dow v. Kaiser Foundation, 90 Cal. Rptr. 747 (1970).
29. See Cobbs v. Grant, *supra* note 10.
30. Canterbury, *supra* note 10.
31. See, for example, American Motorcycle Association v. Davids, 158 N.W. 2d 72 (Mich. App. Ct. 1968); People of the City of Adrian v. Poucher, 247 N.W. 2d 798 (Mich. 1976).
32. See, for example, Application of the President and Directors of Georgetown College, Inc., 331 F. 2d 1000 (D.C. Cir. 1964), cert. den., 377 U.S. 978 (1964); In re Brooks Estate, 205 N.E. 2d 435 (Ill. 1965).
33. Scott v. Bradford, 606 P. 2d 554 (Okla. 1979).
34. Canterbury, *supra* note 10.
35. Cardozo, B. *The Nature of the Judicial Process* (New Haven: Yale University Press, 1921), p. 35.
36. Scott, *supra* note 33.
37. Collins v. Meeker, 424 P. 2d 490 (Kan. 1967).
38. Davis, E. "Canterbury v. Spence et al.—and Informed Consent, Revisited, Three Years Later," 11 *Forum* 708 (1976).
39. Cobbs v. Grant, *supra* note 10.
40. Bly v. Rhoads, 222 S.E. 2d 783 (Va. 1976).
41. Woolley v. Henderson, 418 A. 2d 1123 (Maine 1980).
42. McMullen v. Vaughan, 227 S.E. 2d 40 (Ga. 1976).
43. Malloy v. Shanahan, 421 A. 2d 803 (Pa. Super. 1980).
44. Scaria v. St. Paul Fire & Marine Ins. Co., 227 N.W. 2d 647 (Wis. 1975).
45. Meisel, A. & Kabnick, L., "Informed Consent to Medical Treatment: An Analysis of Recent Legislation," 41 *University of Pittsburgh Law Review* 407 (1980).
46. See, for example, Pa. Health Care Services, Title 40 (Insurance), Section 1301. 103 (1975).
47. See, for example, Neb. Hospital-Malpractice Liability Act, Section 44-2816 (1976).
48. See, for example, Louisiana Public Health & Safety Code, Section 40: 1299.40 (1975).
49. Salgo, *supra* note 12.
50. Katz, *supra* note 13.

Chapter 4

1. Berlin, I., "Two Concepts of Liberty." In *Four Essays on Liberty* (Oxford: Oxford University Press, 1969), pp. 155–156, 158.
2. Hughes, E., "Professions," 92 *Daedalus* 655 (1963).
3. Parsons, T., "The Sick Role and the Role of the Physician Reconsidered," 53 *Milbank Memorial Fund Quarterly* 257 (1975).
4. Garceau, O., *The Political Life of the AMA* (Cambridge: Harvard University Press, 1941), p. 186.
5. See, for example, Goode, W., "Encroachment, Charlatanism, and the Emerging Profession: Psychology, Sociology and Medicine," Presidential Address read at the Annual Meeting of the Eastern Sociological Society, Boston, April, 1960: Reprinted in 25 *American Sociological Review* 902 (1960).
6. Becker, H., "The Nature of a Profession," in *The Sixty-First Yearbook of the National Society for the Study of Education* (Chicago: The National Society for the Study of Education, 1962).
7. See, for example, Parsons, T., *The Social System* (New York: Free Press of Glencoe, 1951), p. 463.
8. See Parsons, T., *supra* note 7; Parsons, T., "A Sociologist Looks at the Legal Profession." In: *Essays in Sociological Theory* (New York: The Free Press of Glencoe, 1954).
9. Parsons, T., *The Social System*, *supra* note 7, at 464–465.
10. According to one version of the Greek myth, Iphigenia was sacrificed to the goddess Artemis by her father Agamemnon. According to another, Iphigenia was rescued from sacrifice by the goddess in the last moment and transported to the land of the Tauri. For my purposes, I have adopted the second version.
11. Pascal, B., *Pensees*, iv. 277.
12. See Sandulescu, "Primum non Nocere: Philological Commentaries on a Medical Aphorism," 13 *Acta Antiqua Hung. Tomus* 359 (1965); Jonsen, A., "Do No Harm: Axiom of Medical Ethics." In: *Philosophical Medical Ethics: Its Nature and Significance*, ed. S. Spicker and H. Engelhardt, Jr. (Dordrecht-Holland: D. Reidel Publishing Company, 1977).
13. *Oath of Hippocrates* (5th century B.C.).
14. See *supra* note 12.
15. Robbins, G., "The Case for Radical Surgery." In: *Breast Cancer Management: Early and Late,* ed. B. Stoll (Chicago: William Heinemann, 1977), pp. 34–35.

16. Freidson, E., *Profession of Medicine* (New York: Dodd, Mead, 1970), p. 336.
17. Burt, R., "Conflict and Trust between Attorney and Client," 69 *Georgetown Law Journal* 1015 (1981).
18. Erikson, E., "Growth and Crises of the 'Healthy Personality.'" In: *Personality in Nature, Society and Culture,* ed. C. Kluckhohn (New York: Alfred A. Knopf, 1955), pp. 185–225.

Chapter 5

1. Beauchamp, T. and Childress, J., *Principles of Biomedical Ethics* (New York: Oxford University Press, 1979), pp. 56–57.
2. Veatch, R., *A Theory of Medical Ethics* (New York: Basic Books, 1981).
3. Kant, I., *Groundwork of the Metaphysic of Morals,* trans. H. Patton (New York: Harper & Row, 1964) p. 80.
4. Cahn, E., "The Lawyer as Scientist and Scoundrel—Reflections on Francis Bacon's Quadricentennial," 36 *New York University Law Review* 1 (1961).
5. Freud, S., "Introductory Lectures on Psycho-Analysis." In: 15 *Standard Edition of the Complete Psychological Works of Sigmund Freud* (London: Hogarth Press, 1963).
6. Hampshire, S., *Two Theories of Morality* (New York: Oxford University Press, 1977), pp. 25–26.
7. Jones, E., 1 *Sigmund Freud: Life and Work* (London: Hogarth Press, 1957), p. 436.
8. Schafer, R., "Regression in the Service of the Ego: The Relevance of a Psychoanalytic Concept for the Personality Assessment." In: *Assessment of Human Motives,* ed. G. Lindzey (New York: Holt, Rinehart and Winston, Inc., 1958), p. 123.
9. Hartmann, H., *Ego Psychology and the Problem of Adaptation,* trans. D. Rapaport (New York: International Universities Press, 1958), p. 72.
10. Loewald, H., *Psychoanalysis and the History of the Individual* (New Haven: Yale University Press, 1978), pp. 15–16, 22.
11. Berlin, I., "Two Concepts of Liberty." In: *Four Essays on Liberty* (Oxford: Oxford University Press, 1969), p. 118.
12. Dworkin, G., "Autonomy and Informed Consent." In: 3 *Making Health Care Decisions* (President's Commission for the Study of Eth-

ical Problems in Medicine and Biomedical and Behavioral Research, 1982), p. 74.

13. Mill, J., *On Liberty* (London: John W. Parker & Son, 1859), pp. 21-23.

14. Middleton, F., "Profile: Richard Selzer," 1 *New Haven Magazine* 37 (July, 1983).

15. Dostoyevsky, F., *The Brothers Karamazov,* trans. D. Magarshack (Baltimore: Penguin Books, 1958), pp. 293, 298-301.

16. Marx, K., "On the Jewish Question." In: 3 *K. Marx and F. Engels: Collected Works* (Moscow: International Publishers, 1974), pp. 162-163.

Chapter 6

1. Blaiberg, P., *Looking at My Heart* (New York: Stein and Day, 1968), pp. 65-66.

2. Fox, R. and Swazey, J., *Courage to Fail* (Chicago: University of Chicago Press, 1974), p. 111.

3. Barnard, C. and Pepper, C., *Christiaan Barnard: One Life* (New York: Macmillan, 1969), pp. 260-61, 360, 392-93.

4. *Webster's New International Dictionary*, Unabridged. 2nd ed. (Springfield, Mass: G. & C. Merriam Company, 1959).

5. Barnard and Pepper, *supra* note 3.

6. Mill, J., *On Liberty* (London: John W. Parker & Son, 1859).

7. Loewald, H., "On the Therapeutic Action of Psychoanalysis." In: *Papers on Psychoanalysis* (New Haven: Yale University Press, 1980), pp. 225-26.

8. Freud, S., "An Autobiographical Study." In: 20 *Standard Edition of the Complete Psychological Works of Sigmund Freud* (London: Hogarth Press, 1959), p. 42.

9. See, generally, Menninger, K., *Theory of Psychoanalytic Technique* (New York: Basic Books, 1958); Orr, D., "Transference and Countertransference: A Historical Survey," 2 *Journal of the American Psychoanalytic Association* 621 (1954); Greenacre, P., "The Role of Transference: Practical Considerations in Relation to Psychoanalytic Therapy," 2 *Journal of the American Psychoanalytic Association* 671 (1954).

10. Freud, S., "An Autobiographical Study," *supra* note 8, p. 42.

11. Freud, A., Unpublished manuscript based on a lecture to students at Case Western Reserve Medical School (October 29, 1964). Re-

printed in Katz, J., *Experimentation with Human Beings* (New York: Russell Sage Foundation, 1972), p. 637.

12. See Berlin, I., *Four Essays on Liberty* (Oxford: Oxford University Press, 1969), p. xxxix.

13. Freud, S., "Observations on Transference—Love." In: 12 *Standard Edition of the Complete Psychological Works of Sigmund Freud* (London: Hogarth Press, 1958).

14. Menninger, R., "Diagnosis of Culture and Social Institutions," 40 *Bulletin of Menninger Clinic* 531 (1976), p. 537.

15. Bird, B., *Talking with Patients* (Philadelphia: J. B. Lippincott, 1973), pp. 14–17.

16. See Loewald, H., *Psychoanalysis and the History of the Individual: The Freud Lectures* (New Haven: Yale University Press, 1978).

17. Loewald, H., "Some Considerations on Repetition and Repetition Compulsion." In: *Papers on Psychoanalysis, supra* note 7, pp. 95–96.

18. Siegler, M., "Critical Illness: The Limits of Autonomy," 7 *Hastings Center Report* 12 (October 1977).

19. Burt, R., *Taking Care of Strangers* (New York: Free Press, 1979).

20. Duff, R. and Hollingshead, A., *Sickness and Society* (New York: Harper & Row, 1968), p. 125.

21. Faden, R. and Faden, A., "False Belief and the Refusal of Medical Treatment," 3 *Journal of Medical Ethics* 133–136 (1977).

22. Aquinas, T., II *Summa Theologica,* Q. 33, 1333–41, trans. Benziger Bros. (1947).

23. Tillich, P., 3 *Systematic Theology* 75 (Chicago: University of Chicago Press, 1963).

24. Oliver, J., "An Ancient Poem on the Duties of a Physician, Part 1," 7 *Bulletin of the History of Medicine* 315 (1939). Reprinted in *Legacies in Ethics and Medicine,* ed. C. Burns (New York: Science History Publications, 1977).

25. Dostoyevsky, F., *The Brothers Karamazov,* trans. D. Magarshack (Baltimore: Penguin Books, 1958), pp. 298–301.

Chapter 7

1. 100 *Gentleman's Magazine* 98 (August, 1830).

2. See, generally, Fox, R., *Experiment Perilous: Physicians and Patients Facing the Unknown* (Glencoe, Ill.: Free Press, 1959); Fox, R. and Swazey, J., *The Courage to Fail: A Social View of Organ Transplants*

and Dialysis (Chicago: University of Chicago Press, 1974 and 1978 [2nd ed.]); Fox, R., "Training for Uncertainty." In: *The Student-Physician,* eds. R. Merton, G. Reader, and P. Kendall (Cambridge: Harvard University Press, 1957), p. 207.

3. Feinstein, A., *Clinical Judgment* (Baltimore: Williams & Wilkins Co., 1967), pp. 23–24.

4. Fox, R., "Training for Uncertainty," *supra* note 2, pp. 208–209.

5. Fox, R., *Experiment Perilous, supra* note 2.

6. Crile, G., Jr., "How Much Surgery for Breast Cancer?" *Modern Medicine* (June 11, 1973), p. 32.

7. Freud, S., "The Interpretation of Dreams," 5 *The Standard Edition of the Complete Psychological Works of Sigmund Freud* (London: Hogarth Press, 1953), p. 499.

8. Dewey, J., *The Quest for Certainty: A Study of the Relation of Knowledge and Action* (New York: Minton, Balch and Company, 1928), pp. 312–313.

9. See generally, Cooper, W., "The History of the Radical Mastectomy," 3 *Annals of Medical History* 36 (1941); Lewison, E., "The History of Breast Cancer and Its Treatment." In: *Breast Cancer and Its Diagnosis and Treatment* (Williams & Wilkins Company, 1955).

10. Lewison, *supra* note 9, p. 17.

11. Halsted, W., "The Results of Operations for the Cure of Cancer of the Breast Performed at the Johns Hopkins Hospital from June, 1889 to January, 1894," 4 *Johns Hopkins Hospital Reports* 297 (1894).

12. Matas, R., "Personal Experience, with Remarks on the Operative Treatment of Cancer of the Breast," 16 *Transactions of the American Surgical Association* 165 (1898).

13. Crile, G., Jr., *A Biologic Consideration of Treatment of Breast Cancer* (Springfield, Ill.: Charles C Thomas, 1967), pp. 41–42.

14. Keynes, G., "Carcinoma of the Breast: An Unorthodox View," *Proceedings of the Cardiff Medical Society* (1954), p. 40.

15. See, for example, Crile, G., Jr., "Management of Breast Cancer: Limited Mastectomy," 230 *Journal of the American Medical Association* 95 (1974); Anglem, T., "Management of Breast Cancer: Radical Mastectomy," 230 *Journal of the American Medical Association* 99 (1974); Crile, G., Jr., "Management of Breast Cancer: Limited Mastectomy in Rebuttal to Dr. Anglem," 230 *Journal of the American Medical Association* 106 (1974).

16. Thomas, L., *The Medusa and the Snail: More Notes of a Biology Watcher* (New York: Viking Press, 1979), pp. 73–74.

17. Thomas, L., "How Should Humans Pay Their Way?" *New York Times* (24 August 1981), p. A15, Columns 2–5.

18. Cope, O., *The Breast* (Boston: Houghton Mifflin Co., 1977), p. 61, 148, 175.

19. See *supra* note 15.

20. Fisher, B. and Wolmack, N., "Systematic Adjuvant (Combined Modality) Therapy in the Treatment of Primary Breast Cancer." In: *Breast Cancer—Advances in Research and Treatment*, ed. W. McGuire (New York: Plenum Medical Book Company, 1977), p. 159.

21. See generally, Moore, F., et al., "Carcinoma of the Breast: A Decade of New Results with Old Concepts," 277 *New England Journal of Medicine* 293, 343, 411, 460 (1967) (Four Parts); Henderson, C. and Canellos, G., "Cancer of the Breast: The Past Decade," 302 New England Journal of Medicine 17, 78 (1980) (Two Parts).

22. Fox, R., "Training for Uncertainty," *supra* note 2.

23. Fox, R., "The Evolution of Medical Uncertainty," 58 *Milbank Memorial Fund Quarterly* 1 (1980), pp. 7–8.

24. Fox, R., "Training for Uncertainty," *supra* note 2.

25. Whitehorn, J., "Education for Uncertainty," 7 *Perspectives in Biology and Medicine* 118 (1963), p. 119.

26. See Fox, R., *The Courage to Fail, supra* note 2.

27. Conant, J., quoted in Fox, R., "Training for Uncertainty," *supra* note 2, p. 207.

28. Knafl, K. and Burkett, G., "Professional Socialization in a Surgical Specialty: Acquiring Medical Judgment," 9 *Social Science and Medicine* 397 (1975).

29. Light, D., Jr., "Uncertainty and Control in Professional Training," 20 *Journal of Health and Social Behavior* 310 (1979), p. 320.

30. Kuhn, T., *The Structure of Scientific Revolutions* (Chicago: University of Chicago Press, 1970) (2nd ed.).

31. Wolf, S., "The Pharmacology of Placebos," 11 *Pharmacological Reviews* 689 (1959). Also see generally, Bok, S., "The Ethics of Giving Placebos," 231 *Scientific American* 17 (1974); Bok, S., *Lying: Moral Choice in Public and Private Life* (New York: Random House, 1978).

32. Remarks of Dr. Dean Hashimoto, then a second year student at Yale Law School.

33. Houston, R., "The Doctor Himself as a Therapeutic Agent," 11 *Annals of Internal Medicine* 1415 (1938), p. 1418.

34. Beecher, H., "Surgery as Placebo," 176 *Journal of the American Medical Association* 1102 (1961).

35. Brody, H., "The Lie that Heals: The Ethics of Giving Placebos," 97 *Annals of Internal Medicine* 112 (1982).

36. Houston, *supra* note 33, p. 1418.

37. Scheff, T., "Decision Rules, Types of Error and Their Consequences in Medical Diagnosis," 8 *Behavioral Science* 97 (1963).

38. Ingelfinger, F., "Arrogance," 303 *New England Journal of Medicine* 1507 (1980), p. 1509.

39. See, for example, Braunwald, E., "Coronary-Artery Surgery at the Crossroads," 297 *New England Journal of Medicine* 661 (1977); McIntosh, H. and Garcia, J., "The First Decade of Aorto-coronary Bypass Grafting, 1967–1977: A Review," 57 *Circulation* 405 (1978); Braunwald, E., "Effects of Coronary-Artery Bypass Grafting on Survival," 309 *New England Journal of Medicine* 1181 (1983).

40. See, for example, Bakwin, H., "Pseudodoxia Pediatrica," 232 *New England Journal of Medicine* 691 (1945).

41. Waitzkin, H. and Stoeckle, J., "The Communication of Information about Illness: Clinical, Sociological, and Methodological Considerations," 8 *Advances in Psychosomatic Medicine* 180 (1972), p. 187–188.

42. Gorovitz, S. and MacIntyre, A., "Toward a Theory of Medical Fallibility," 1 *Journal of Medicine and Philosophy* 51 (1976).

43. *Modern Medicine,* W. Osler and T. McCrae eds. (New York: Lea Bros. & Co., 1907), p. xxxi.

44. Forman, M., *The Letters of John Keats* (London: Oxford University Press, 1931), p. 72.

45. Trilling, L., *The Opposing Self* (New York: Viking Press, 1955), p. 35.

46. Keats, J., "Ode on a Grecian Urn." In: *The Major Poets: English and American,* C. Coffin ed. (New York: Harcourt, Brace & World, 1954).

47. Trilling, *supra* note 45, p. 37.

48. Whitehorn, *supra* note 25, p. 122.

49. Forman, *supra* note 44.

50. Oliver, J., "An Ancient Poem on the Duties of a Physician, Part 1," 7 *Bulletin of the History of Medicine* 315 (1939). Reprinted in: *Legacies in Ethics and Medicine,* ed. C. Burns (New York: Science History Publications, 1977).

51. Proust, M., "The Guermantes Way." In: 2 *Remembrance of Things Past,* trans. C. Moncrieff and T. Kilmartin (New York: Random House, 1981), p. 308.

Chapter 8

1. Code of Ethics of the American Medical Association (adopted May, 1847), Chapter 1, Article II, Section 3.
2. Parsons, T., *The Social System* (New York: Free Press of Glencoe, 1951), p. 463.
3. Cassel, E., "The Nature of Suffering and the Goals of Medicine," 306 *New England Journal of Medicine* 639 (1982).
4. See, for example, Weisman, A. and Hackett, T., "Predilection to Death: Death and Dying as a Psychiatric Problem," 23 *Psychosomatic Medicine* 232 (1961).
5. The absence of such data is noted in McIntosh, J., "Processes of Communication, Information Seeking and Control Associated with Cancer: A Selective Review of the Literature," 8 *Social Science and Medicine* 167 (1974). Also see Veatch, R., *Death, Dying and the Biological Revolution* (New Haven: Yale University Press, 1976); Glaser, B. and Strauss, A., *Awareness of Dying* (Chicago: Aldine Publishing Company, 1965).
6. Veatch, R., *supra* note 5, p. 237.
7. Shneidman, E., "Suicide." In: *Taboo Topics,* ed. N. Farberow (New York: Atherton Press, 1963).
8. Freud, S., "Thoughts for the Times on War and Death," 14 *Standard Edition of the Complete Psychological Works of Sigmund Freud* (London: Hogarth Press, 1957), p. 289.
9. Becker, E., *The Denial of Death* (New York: Free Press, 1973), p. ix.
10. James, W., *Varieties of Religious Experiences: A Study in Human Nature* (New York: Mentor Edition, 1958), p. 121.
11. Becker, *supra* note 9, pp. 26–27.
12. Freud, *supra* note 8, p. 299.
13. Feifel, H., et al., "Physicians Consider Death," *Proceedings of the American Psychological Association* 201 (1967).
14. See, for example, Oken, D., "What to Tell Cancer Patients," 175 *Journal of the American Medical Association* 1120 (1961).
15. Acts 5, 1:2.

16. Cannon, W., "Voodoo Death," 19 *Psychosomatic Medicine* 170 (1957).

17. Milton, G., "Self-Willed Death or the Bone Pointing Syndrome," *Lancet* (June 23, 1973), p. 1435; Gillin, J., "Magical Fright," 11 *Psychiatry* 387 (1948).

18. See, for example, Weisman and Hackett, *supra* note 4.

19. Paul, O. and Schatz, M., "On Sudden Death," 43 *Circulation* 7 (1971). See also Engel, G., "Psychologic Factors in Instantaneous Cardiac Death," 294 *New England Journal of Medicine* 664 (1976).

20. Barber, T., "Death by Suggestion," 23 *Psychosomatic Medicine* 153 (1961).

21. Weisman and Hackett, *supra* note 4, p. 255.

22. Thomas, D., "Do not go gentle into that good night." In: *Poems of Dylan Thomas* (New York: New Directions Publishing Corporation, 1952).

23. Cabot, R., "The Use of Truth and Falsehood in Medicine," 5 *American Medicine* 344 (1903). Reprinted in *Ethics in Medicine: Historical Perspectives and Contemporary Concerns,* ed. S. Reiser, A. Dyck and W. Curran (Cambridge, Mass.: Massachusetts Institute of Technology Press, 1977).

24. Hackett, T. and Weisman, A., "When to Tell Dying Patients the Truth," *Medical Economics* 81 (4 December 1961).

Index

255